December 2005.

To Brian + Mona.

With all best wishes.

Joan and Jenny.

LIFE'S JIGSAW:
A MEDICAL MAN
FINDS THE PIECES

Life's Jigsaw: A Medical Man Finds the Pieces

by

JOHN RICHMOND
CBE, MD, FRCPE, FRCP, FRSE

Emeritus Professor of Medicine
University of Sheffield and
Past President Royal College
of Physicians of Edinburgh

The Memoir Club

© John Richmond 2001

First published in 2001 by
The Memoir Club
Whitworth Hall
Spennymoor
County Durham

British Library Cataloguing in
Publication Data.
A catalogue record for this book
is available from the
British Library.

ISBN: 1 84104 025 8

Typeset by George Wishart & Associates, Whitley Bay.
Printed by Bookcraft (Bath) Ltd.

To Jenny

Contents

Illustrations

Foreword

IF WALTON HIMSELF WAS *The Compleat Angler*, read on and judge whether this biography was written by a man who might well be regarded as *The Compleat Physician* . . . because John Richmond has served with distinction in so many of the fields of Medicine.

He was assuredly held in high regard as a family doctor in Whithorn. Before that, he acquired a truly outstanding range and quality of experience as a (National Service) Army Doctor in Africa. He went on to be a most successful hospital physician and was successively Lecturer, Senior Lecturer and Reader in Medicine at Edinburgh. And he then proceeded to embellish the Chair of Medicine at Sheffield, taking the Deanship there in his stride and with prestigious senior status accorded to him in the London College of Physicians. He returned to Edinburgh where his term as President of the Royal College of Physicians of Edinburgh was a great success. It is a pleasure to write a foreword to this all-too-brief biography of a remarkable man who has been my close friend for forty eventful years. The challenge is to do justice to his character without overindulgence in superlatives, because my admiration will be obvious.

John's personal account in the following pages reflects much of his typically guarded understatement. But his readers cannot fail to be impressed by his record of so much achievement and his daunting combination of industry, determination and great ability. His patients, his friends, his colleagues, his guests and his students will all testify to the constancy of his authority, his courtesy, his gentleness, his unyielding integrity and his strength. I have cast this paragraph almost as a reference, because the style of the biography is unassuming but these points must be made.

Here is the story of a dedicated doctor, a gifted teacher and a man of uncompromising honesty who has never lost his friendly nature, his warmth and his human touch. These qualities have survived, despite the need (increasingly evident in these difficult years) for the determined competitiveness that he displayed in sport – in his swimming and diving, and on the rugby field – and in his very successful academic studies. He has also been able to develop and display firmness and to hold to his high principles in his teaching, his clinical management, and notably in his senior committee work. He makes light of his courageous responses to many of the very demanding challenges that he faced. And he sprinkles his biography nicely with anecdotes that reveal his grand sense of humour and love of good stories. He is, himself, an accomplished raconteur.

John Richmond has won the acclaim and unreserved respect of his professional colleagues across the world for his outstanding contributions to Medicine and to medical education at undergraduate and postgraduate levels. He holds many honours. His personal friends will warm to his many fine tributes to Jenny, his wife, and they will join me in applauding this modest chronicle of his remarkable career.

Gerald Collee
(Emeritus Professor of Medical Microbiology, University of Edinburgh)
Edinburgh 2001

Preface

IT IS AN HONOUR, but also somewhat embarrassing, to be approached with the invitation to write one's memoirs. I demurred two or three times but eventually, with some trepidation, decided to proceed. The main concern was that it might all read like self-aggrandisement, which is the last thing that I would want to happen. Also I had to wonder who would be interested apart from family, close friends and colleagues.

There is quite a lot about climbing the ladder in teaching hospital and postgraduate medicine and about doors opening unexpectedly. However I have tried to pepper the story with happy memories, anecdotes and my enjoyment of humour. There are many quotations and while the odd word may have changed with the passage of time, I am sure that the content is close to the original; indeed, I can still hear the voices.

I have purposely not mentioned many friends and colleagues by name and I sincerely hope that no one will be offended by any significant omission of a piece of the jigsaw.

Finally I want to thank my good friend Gerald Collee for his extraordinarily generous Foreword and also the many staff of the Memoir Club who have given me so much help and encouragement.

Acknowledgements

1. The Richmond Surname Society.
2. The Head Teacher, Hall Cross School, Doncaster, formerly Doncaster Grammar School.
3. Air Images, Haltwhistle, Northumberland NE49 0DG.
4. Blackwell Science Ltd.
5. President and Council, Royal College of Physicians of Edinburgh.
6. *A History of the Royal College of Physicians of London*, Vol I, by Sir George Clark, Clarendon Press, Oxford, for the Royal College of Physicians 1964.
7. The Medical Pilgrims.
8. The Public Relations Office, University of Sheffield.
9. Emeritus Professor Donald H. Girdwood.
10. 'Bicentenary of the Faculty of Medicine 1726-1926' by University of Edinburgh.

CHAPTER 1

Origins and Early Childhood, 1926-36

THE FAMILY NAME 'Richmond' is believed to have
originated in the eleventh century. It may be derived
from 'Riche-monte' meaning fine or noble hill, of which
there were many in northern France. It was a splendid term
for the Richmond Castle site in North Yorkshire on the
River Swale.

The first Constable of Richmond Castle was Rhasculpus
Musard de Richemont born in 1070, his father being
Roaldus Musard de Richemonde born in 1028, and the
surname may have evolved from that time. One particular
family tree has been traced right back to that period. After
Rhasculpus the name Musard seems to have been abandoned
but 'de Richmonte' continued until the fourteenth century
when in succeeding generations it became Rychemonde,
Rycheman, Richman and finally a John Richmond was born
in 1561. Another fascinating feature of this particular family
pedigree is that Oliffe Richmond was born in 1881; he
became Professor of Humanity in the University of
Edinburgh and actually 'capped' me at my own graduation.

There are Richmonds all over the world and of course
there could be many sources of the name other than North
Yorkshire. My own family goes back for many generations in
Ayrshire, Scotland. Indeed one of Robert Burns's best
friends was a John Richmond, but I cannot claim any direct
connection.

My father was born in 1899 and might have been caught up in the First World War had he not been plagued with the asthma/eczema syndrome from infancy. His own father, John Richmond, had gained a Colliery Manager's Certificate in Glasgow and moved the family to Larkhall, Lanarkshire in 1912 when he became General Manager of a group of collieries in south Lanarkshire owned by the Darngavil Coal Company. The collieries were to be mostly 'worked out' by the late 1930s and early 1940s, but this background is possibly why my father took a BSc in mining engineering at Glasgow University. In 1923 he migrated to Doncaster in South Yorkshire to start a Department of Mining in the College of Technology. I believe that the original thirty students studying for various coal mining certificates was later to increase in number to around 600 because of the great expansion and importance of the South Yorkshire coalfield. Father was later to become Principal of a very large College which had grown to embrace many disciplines.

He married Janet Hyslop Brown in 1924, also from Larkhall and daughter of James Brown the Gas Manager. While my father had four sisters, my mother's mother had died at her birth and she had been brought up by her father and a maiden aunt.

I was born on 30 May 1926. It is not a particularly notable anniversary although Joan of Arc was burned at the stake on 30 May. I was to grow up in a nice friendly area, Wheatley Hills, on the eastern outskirts of Doncaster. Then it was next to open farming country and there were two nearby golf courses. Indeed, I can recall in the 1930s peeping through the hedge bordering one of the golf courses, watching a slightly disabled man who was playing. Then I

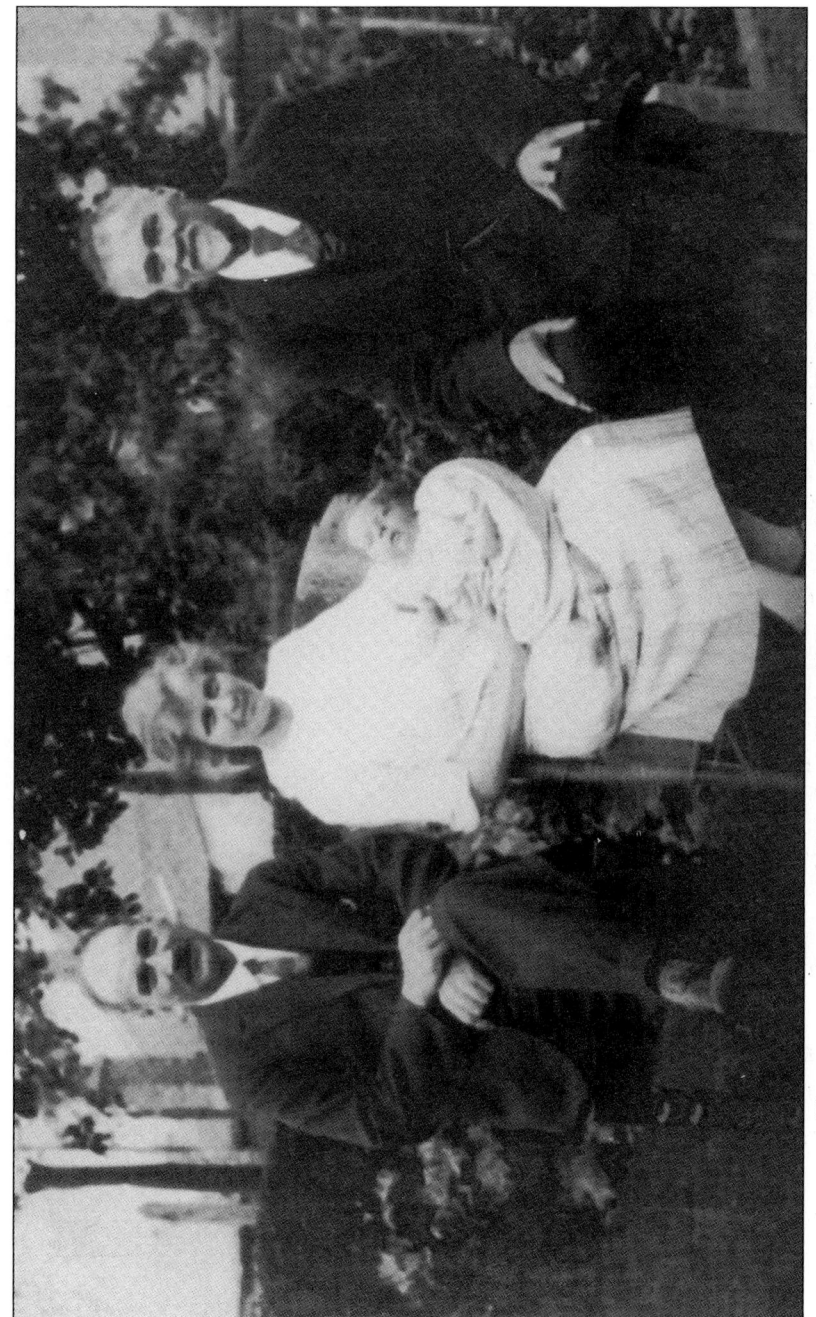

Four generations with Mother, Grandfather and Great-grandfather Brown.

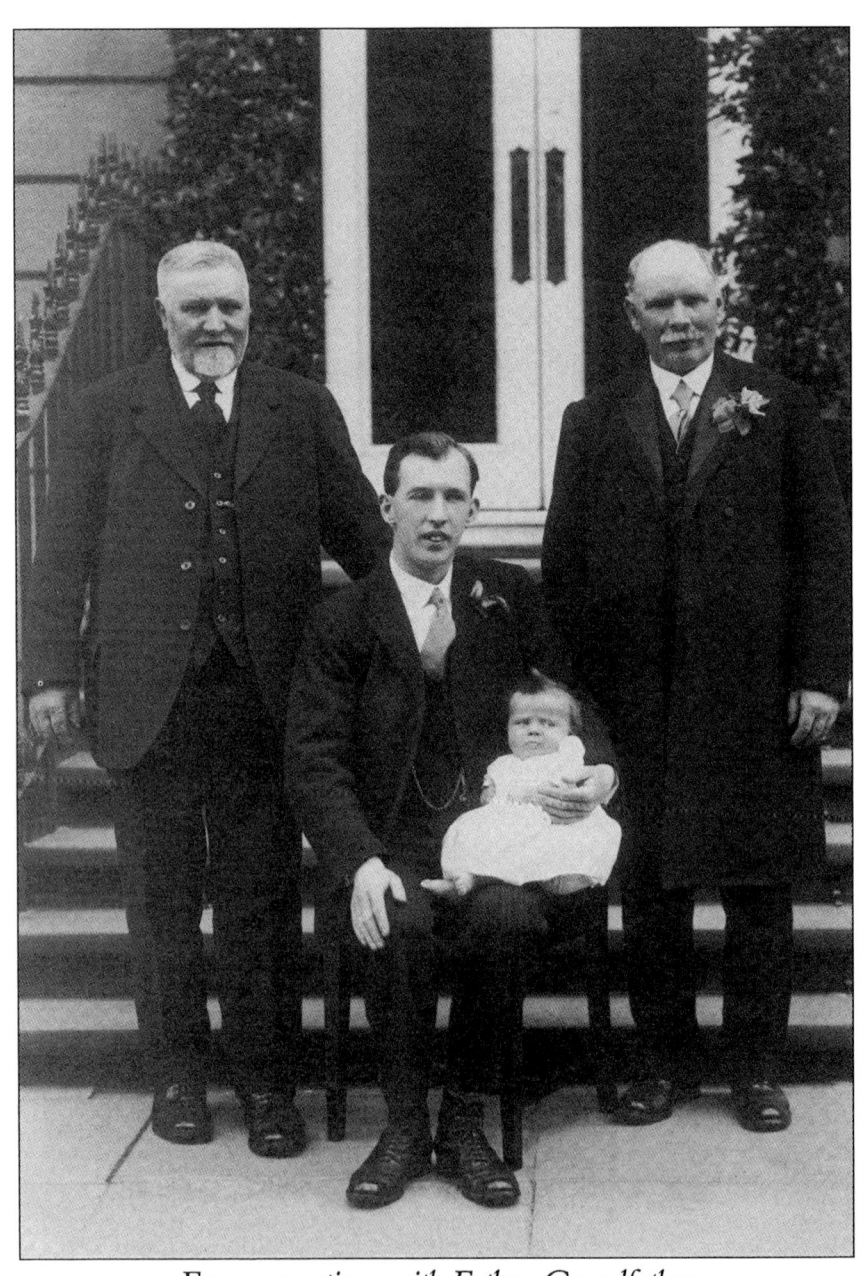

*Four generations with Father, Grandfather
and Great-grandfather Richmond.*

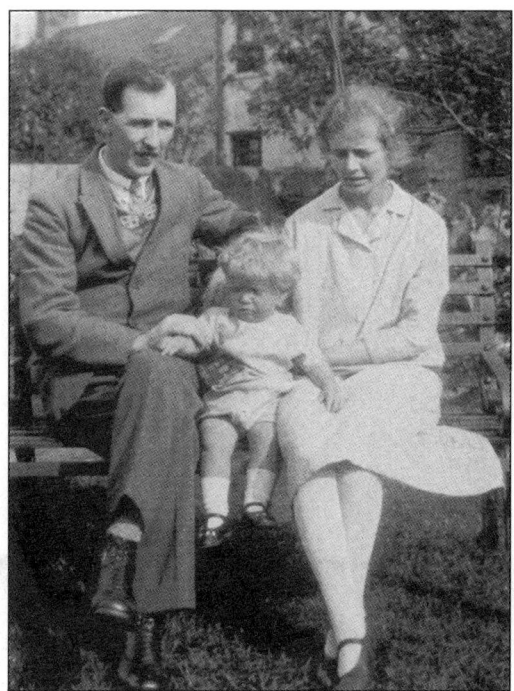

With parents in garden of Richmond
grandparents in Larkhall, summer 1927.

was most surprised to see him knock out his pipe on one of his artificial legs; it was the great Douglas Bader.

An old stone quarry in the area was converted into a lovely boating lake which reminds me of an early addiction to Yorkshire humour. It was rumoured that at a meeting of the Town Council, a Councillor had proposed that it would be a good idea to put a gondola on the lake, and then one of his colleagues went on to suggest that they should have two and then they could 'breed off 'em'!

Schooling started early in 1931 when I was still aged four, at the new Intake Junior Mixed School. It was in fact a primary and junior school. 'Mixed' was a good adjective

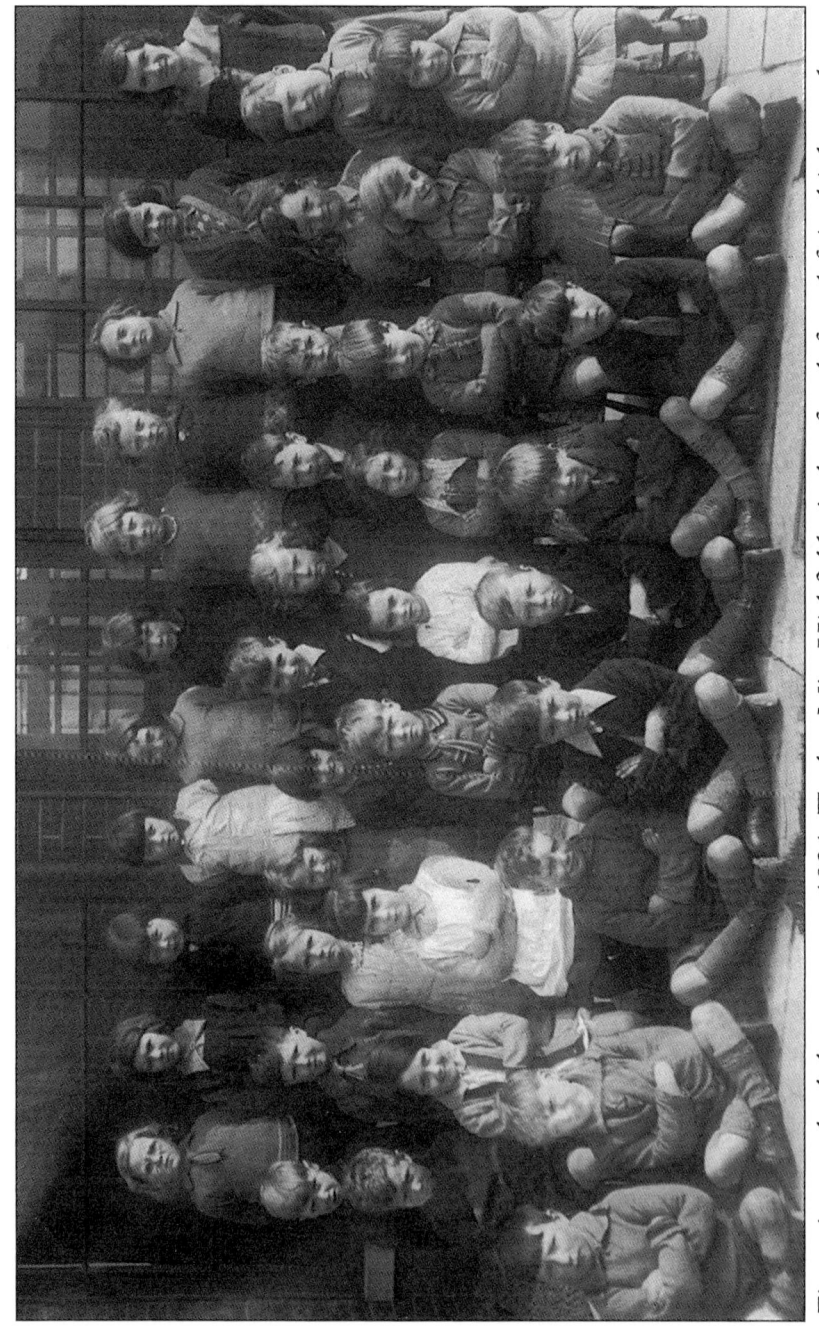

First primary school class, summer 1931. Teacher Miss Highfield. Author fourth from left in third row down.

because while it was in the middle of a large council estate near the racecourse it drained a wide area and the social mix was splendid. Although the Head Teacher was a delightful man, nearly all the teachers were women and they were outstanding.

In my first few days I was greatly moved by the morning assembly conducted by the Head Teacher. We all had to recite together the Lord's Prayer, but the young at the front had to pick up the words from the older children in the rows behind. My parents were delighted to hear about the Lord's Prayer but were not impressed when I gave them my first version; 'Our Father who shot in Heaven, Harold be thy name . . .'

We were in A and B streams in the junior school, by which time the average class size was fifty pupils, seated in serried ranks, something which would be unacceptable today. Another recollection is that from an early age I cycled solo from home to school through a field and the fringe of a sand quarry 2 miles to and fro', including lunch time. This might cause concern today.

Apart from schooling it was a happy childhood, in which I was joined after a few years by a brother and then after a further few years by a sister. With my father being in education we had generous family holidays in the summer, usually at some sea resort and ending up with the relatives in Larkhall. Sadly my maternal grandfather died in 1932 in his fifties. It was then the custom in Scotland that the coffin would be lowered into the grave by the nearest eight relatives and friends, the closest taking the cord at the head. At the age of six I was the senior mourner on my mother's side and having led the cortege behind the horse-drawn hearse to the cemetery, I had to take the head of grand-

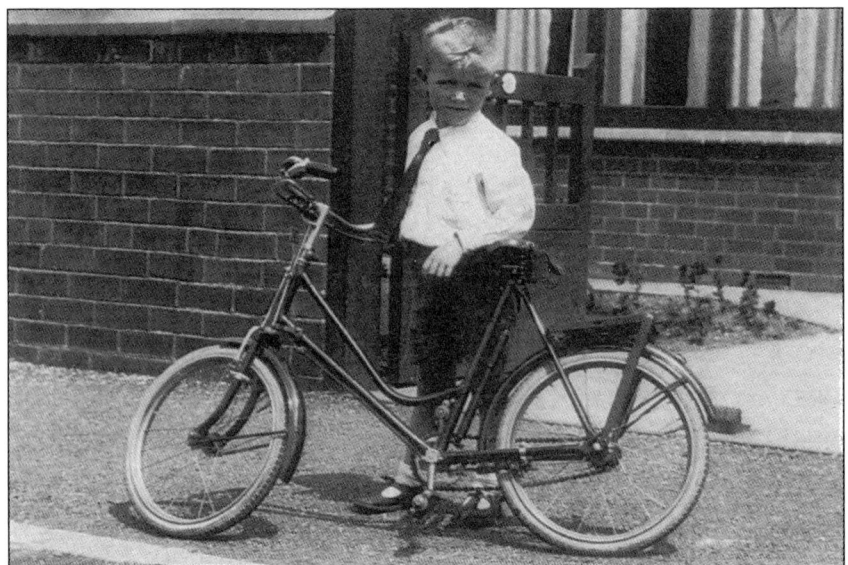

*The first bicycle for school. From 1932 I would
travel approximately eight miles per day.*

father Brown's coffin, assisted by grandfather Richmond.
I had to do the same two years later when the maiden
aunt died. These were memorable events that have left no
scars.

Around this time in Doncaster we were fortunate to have
an outstanding Secretary to the Education Committee, Mr
Danby. Through him a programme of weekly swimming
lessons was started for all junior school children at the
Corporation Swimming Baths. I obtained my first certificate
for swimming one length and then three lengths in 1935,
and through this initiation, swimming was to become a
major sporting interest in later years.

Having mentioned the Lord's Prayer, I should mention
that my childhood was in a strict and deeply religious home.
My parents had been brought up in the Plymouth Brethren,

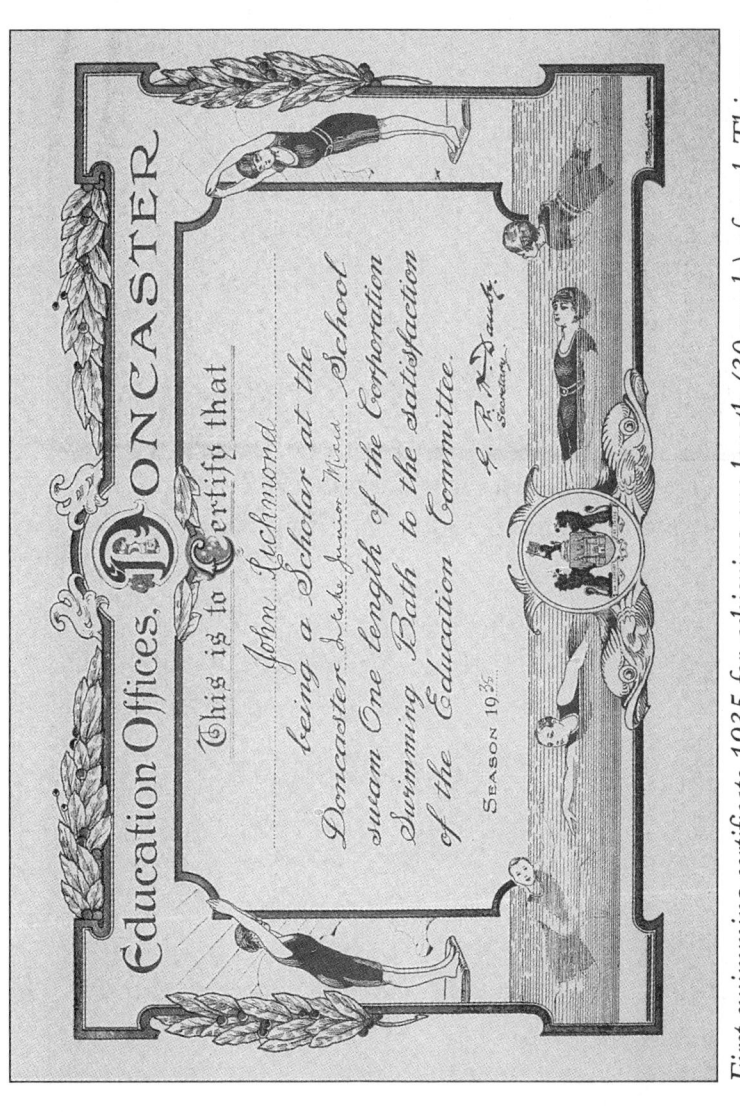

First swimming certificate 1935 for achieving one length (30 yards) of pool. This was followed a few weeks later by a second certificate for three lengths by different strokes, one to be backstroke. A life-long interest followed.

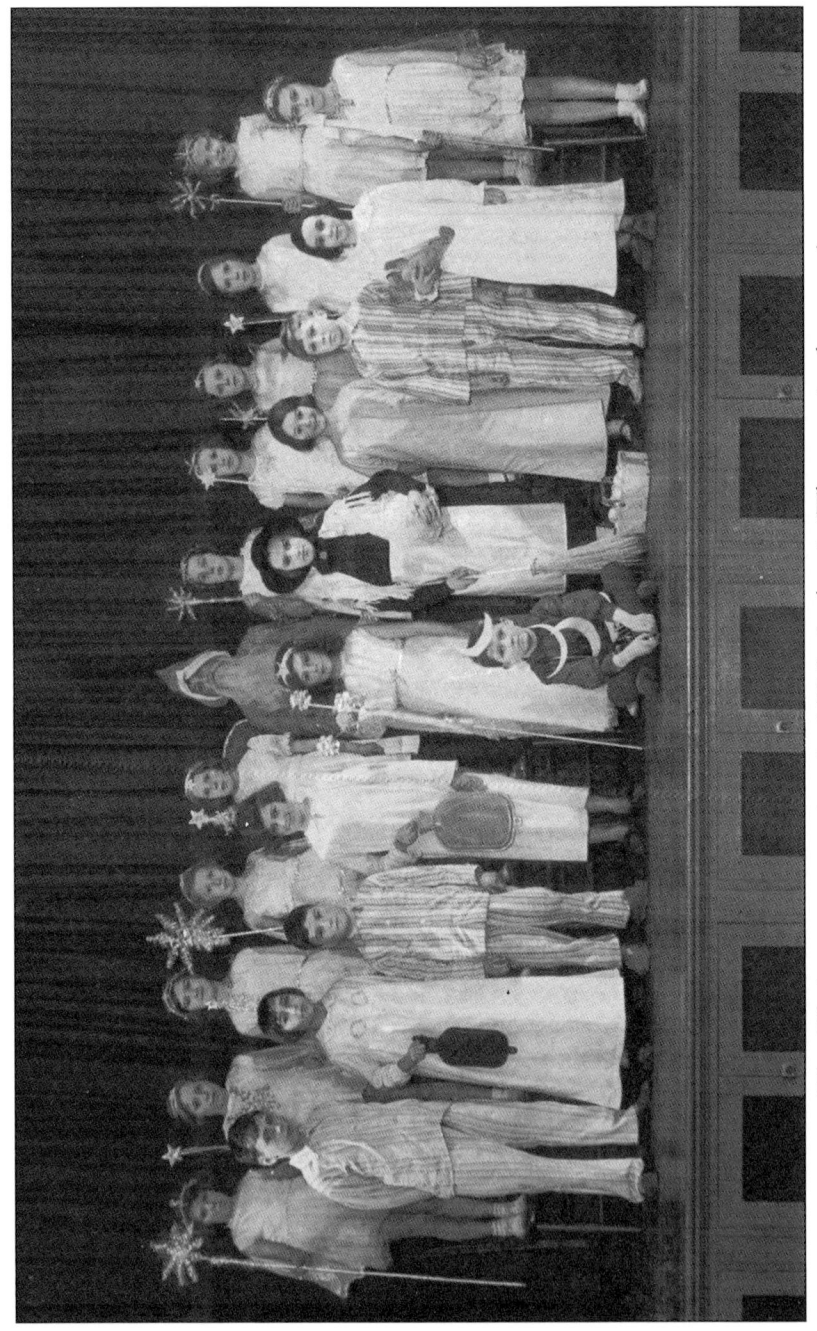

The Christmas pantomime in 1935. Author is 'The man in the moon'.

which was very strong in the west of Scotland. I still greatly enjoy hearing rousing gospel hymns. Also in 1935 we went for the first time to the cinema because my parents were particularly keen to see King George V's funeral on Pathé News. My mother was convulsed with laughter during the main film, Laurel and Hardy in *Bonnie Scotland*, and things were never quite the same again.

What came next was to begin the shaping of my whole career. In Doncaster then, children around ten and eleven years of age sat the 'Scholarship Examination' in the spring of the last year at the junior school. This would be the precursor of the 'Eleven +'. For reasons not very clear, a few of us in form 3A, the penultimate year, were allowed to take the examination a year early. I was only nine years old, shortly to be ten, and to my surprise I passed. Also in those days there was streaming into the secondary schools. The boys who passed the examination went to Doncaster Grammar School, and the girls to the Girls' High School. Depending on examination performance, a second group went to the Central School where they followed a similar curriculum and from where it was possible to gain promotion to the Grammar School or High School if there was later academic improvement. The third group went to my father's college where there was available a wide range of training, not only in the 'three R's', but also in technical skills for the boys, and for the girls, an introduction to other subjects such as domestic science and secretarial work. While the fourth group did have comprehensive schooling one can imagine that these children may have found it more difficult than the children in the other groups to go on to the next stage.

Over the years, primary and secondary education has

been the subject of much change and controversy and the debate for and against early streaming and selection still continues.

CHAPTER 2

Doncaster Grammar School, 1936-43

DONCASTER GRAMMAR SCHOOL was a boy's school with long-standing traditions. In recent years it has become a comprehensive co-educational school known as Hall Cross School. However the Grammar School was recently able to celebrate its 650th anniversary having had its first mention in the time of Edward III in the York Chapter Act Book of 19 May 1350.

I cannot praise enough the dedicated schoolmasters who followed the grand teachers of the previous school. Indeed many of the attitudes and values I now have were absorbed from these men. The same social mix continued.

Again I have many happy memories and select a few from my second year. One was a most detailed and informative trip to London by train and then a coach tour, which took in most of the sights. In the summer of 1938 a group was taken to Headingly to watch the Fourth Test Match against Australia and spent the day sitting on the grass just outside the boundary. The many well-known figures on the field included Hammond, Verity, Fleetwood-Smith, Farnes and O'Reilly, although the outstanding event was the innings of Don Bradman, 103 not out. But I need to add one other occasion, the swimming contest against Barnsley Grammar School. At the risk of sounding immodest, I won the diving event and then was awarded my Half-Colours for swimming, in the bus on the way home!

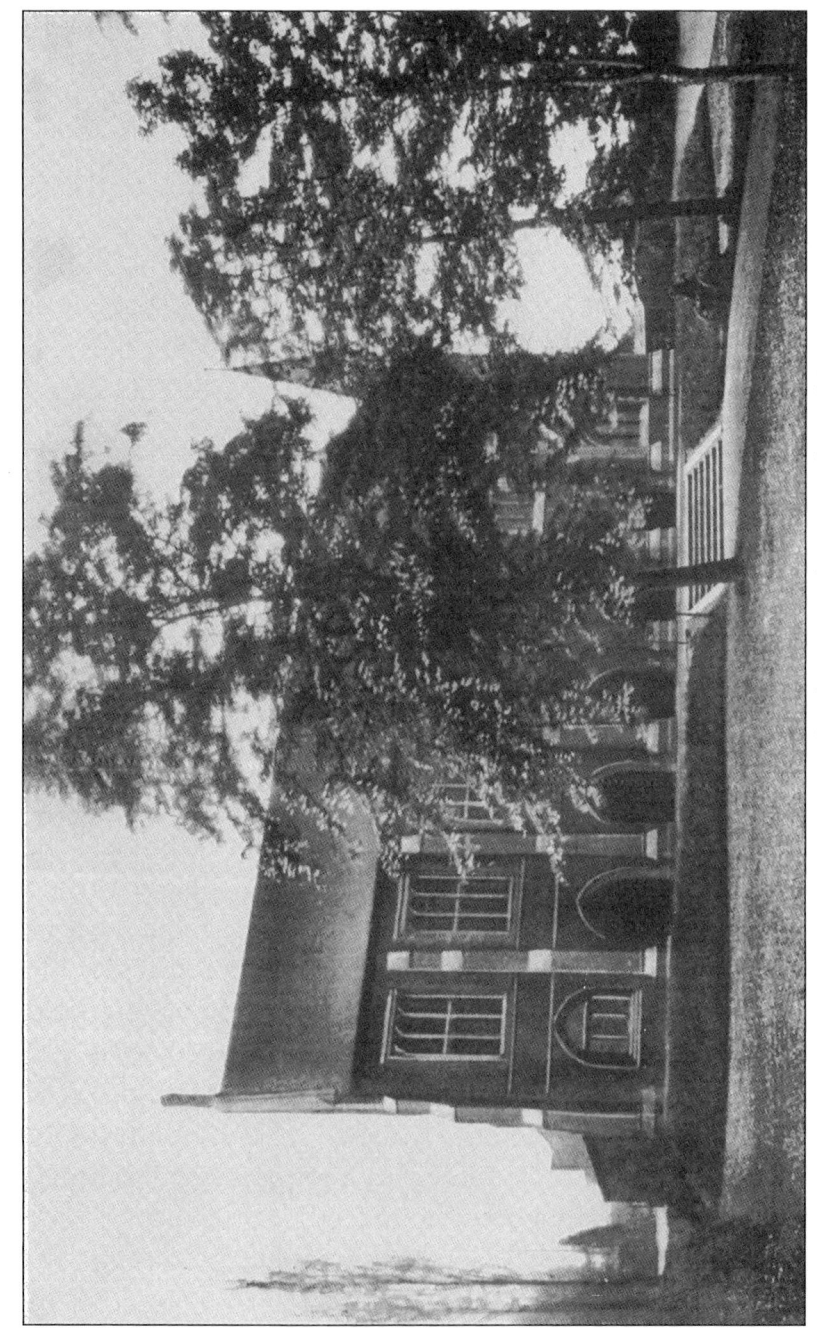

Doncaster Grammar School prior to the Second World War.

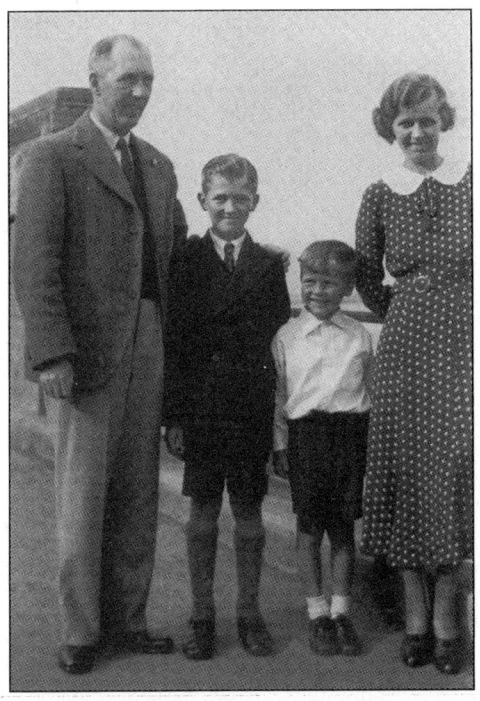

With parents and younger brother James in 1937.

Some rather critical academic landmarks followed. At the end of the 3rd year (now aged thirteen) we had to decide between the subjects of German, Greek and Chemistry. I do not recall seeking any advice but Chemistry it had to be. This was when the Second World War was about to begin. Then in the summer term of the 5th year (now aged fourteen and soon to be fifteen) we sat the School Certificate Examination, the present equivalent being 'O' Levels and GCSEs. Like the rest of my class I took nine subjects with pleasing results.

I had many good pals at this time not only in the school but also among neighbours. Looking at a photograph of Form 5A (the School Certificate Year) some of the boys

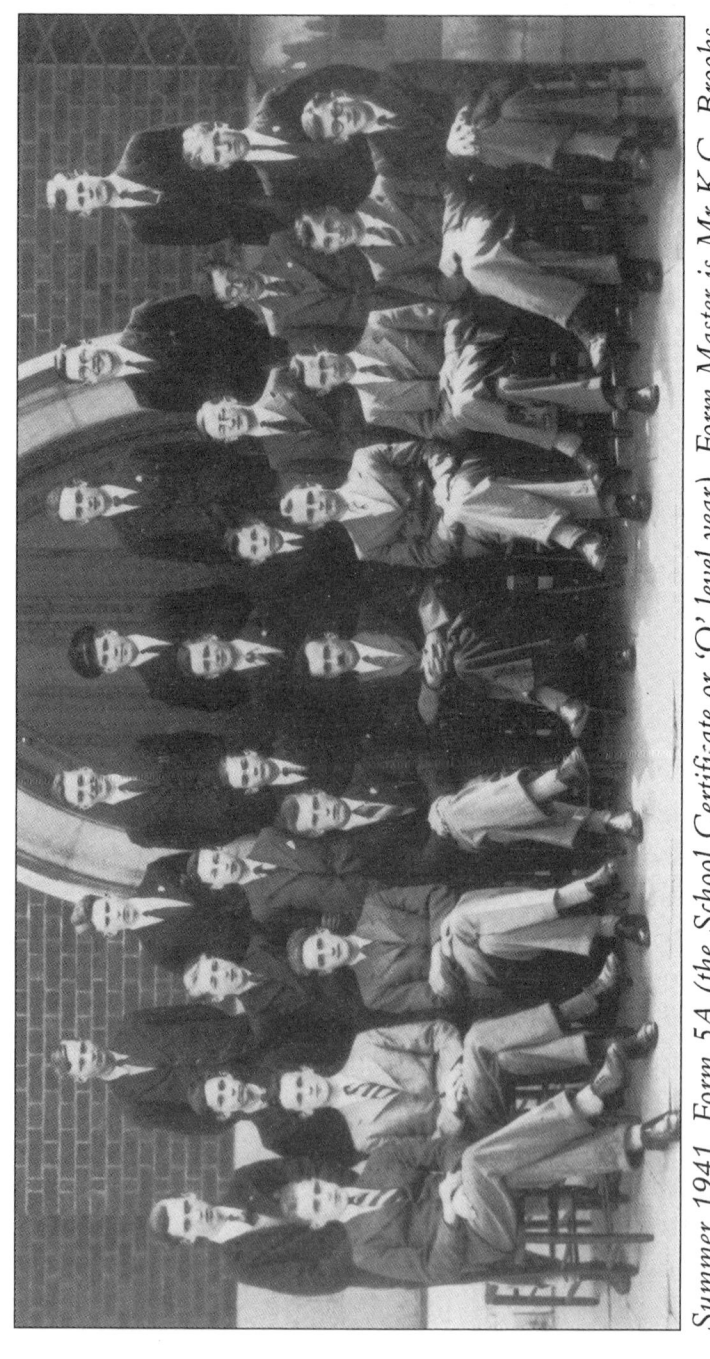

Summer 1941. Form 5A (the School Certificate or 'O' level year). Form Master is Mr K.G. Brooks. Author is at right-hand end of second row. The classmate in uniform in back row had just joined the Merchant Navy. The late Sir Roy Watts is on Mr Brooks's right. Because of wartime clothing restrictions we are not all in school uniform.

appear a little older then fifteen and sixteen. One dear friend was the late Sir Roy Watts, one-time Chief Executive of BEA, then British Airways, then head of Thames Water. He was an outstanding cricketer and rugby player but most of us enjoyed sport and I myself was honoured with Colours in rugby (scrum-half), athletics and, of course, swimming. The swimming included getting the cup as Junior Swimming Champion and then Senior Swimming Champion.

In 1938-40, the school was rebuilt, but retaining the old library and cloisters and apart from excellent new class-rooms, laboratories, gymnasium and swimming pool we now had a squash court and a fives court, and of course ready access to the adjacent playing fields on Town Moor. I also recall many schoolmasters devoting themselves to out-of-hours activities, which apart from sport included a scout troop and a very enthusiastic choir. The choir got as far as performing the whole of Handel's *Messiah* in public to great acclaim.

Because of the war we used to take it in turns in groups to 'fire watch', supervised by a schoolmaster, in the tower of the new school. My group used to drink large volumes of cider, apparently without realising that cider contained quite a lot of alcohol. We also had, compulsorily, to join the Air Training Corps in the 5th and 6th Forms. Apart from regular drill sessions we had interesting visits to local RAF stations and these included some short flights in warplane cockpits.

In my last year in 1942-3, I was enormously honoured to be made School Captain and enjoyed the loyalty and support of seven other prefects. One punishment comes into my mind, which has certainly changed in recent years. The cane was used by the masters from time to time, sometimes for very minor offences, and no one seemed to object. I myself

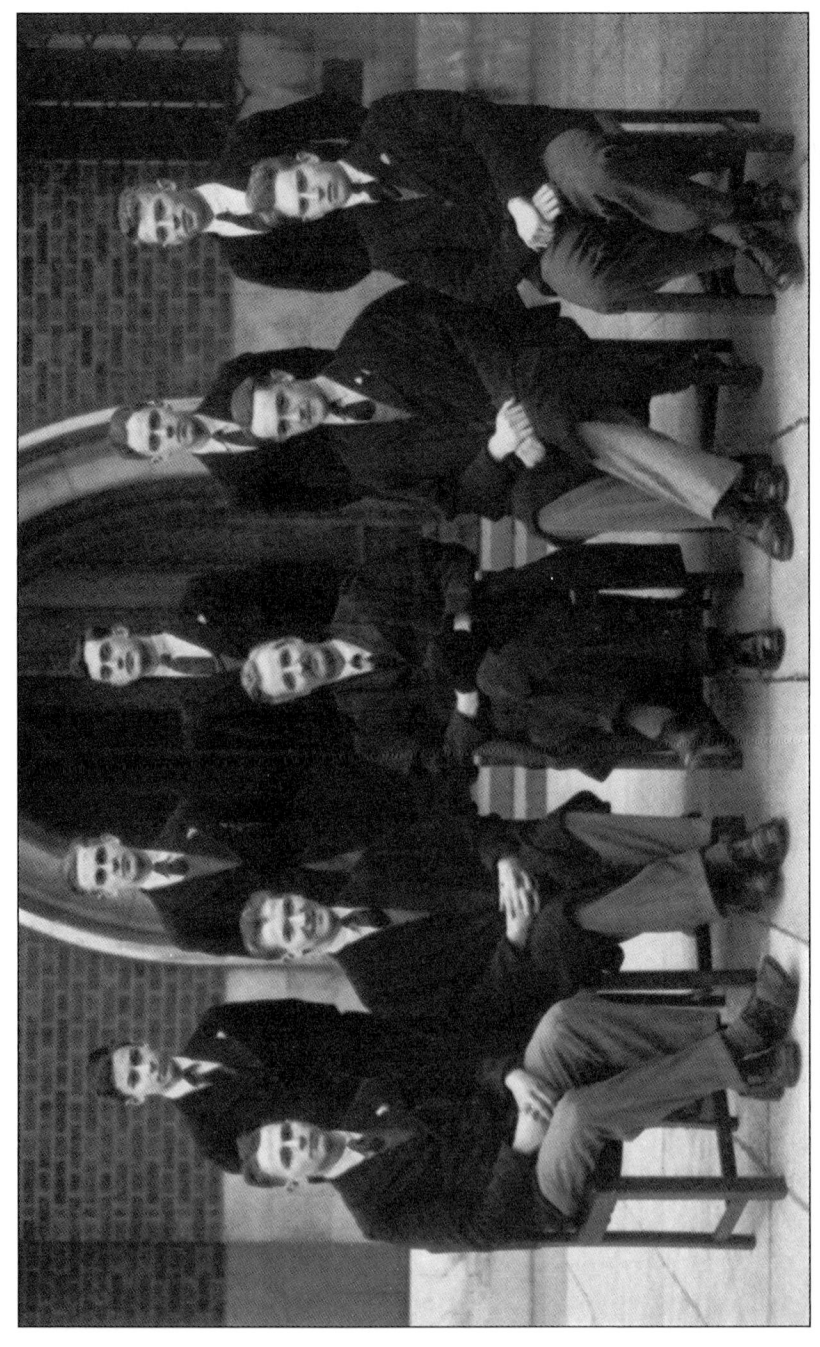

Summer 1943. The prefects with Headmaster Mr F.C. Lay. Author is on Mr Lay's right.

had four painful strokes on the 'derrière', on one occasion for 'talking'. Prefects were also allowed to give bad boys the slipper in the School Captain's room, and they did, albeit with constraint.

The new school hall was very effectively blacked out in the war period. Because of this the Council for the Encouragement of Music and the Arts (CEMA), used the hall quite extensively for concerts. These included one by part of the London Philharmonic Orchestra but I recall particularly the many pianists who came, including Myra Hess, Benno Moiseiwitsch, Pouischnoff and Nina Milkina. When Mark Hambourg came from Leeds I happened to have been put in charge of the lights in the wings of the stage. His recital included *The Moonlight Sonata*, which I had learned to play myself. Those who know the piece will remember that the left hand is mostly octave chords but Mr Hambourg seemed to have all five fingers busy for most of the time. When he came off the stage mopping his brow, I said to him rather impertinently, 'Excuse me, sir, which edition were you playing from?' to which he replied, 'I was playing it just as Beethoven would have liked it, lad'!

I was now approaching Higher School Certificate (now 'A' Levels) in which my subjects would be Chemistry, Physics and Mathematics with subsidiary Biology. In retrospect it seems most inappropriate that our general secondary education in English, History, Geography, Latin, French and Art had to be left behind at such a young age; I was only just fifteen. The same is true today, whereas in Scotland, a somewhat broader band of subjects tends to be taken in Scottish Highers, up to the point of leaving school.

One sad embarrassment remains as I conclude my memories of Doncaster Grammar School. I do not know

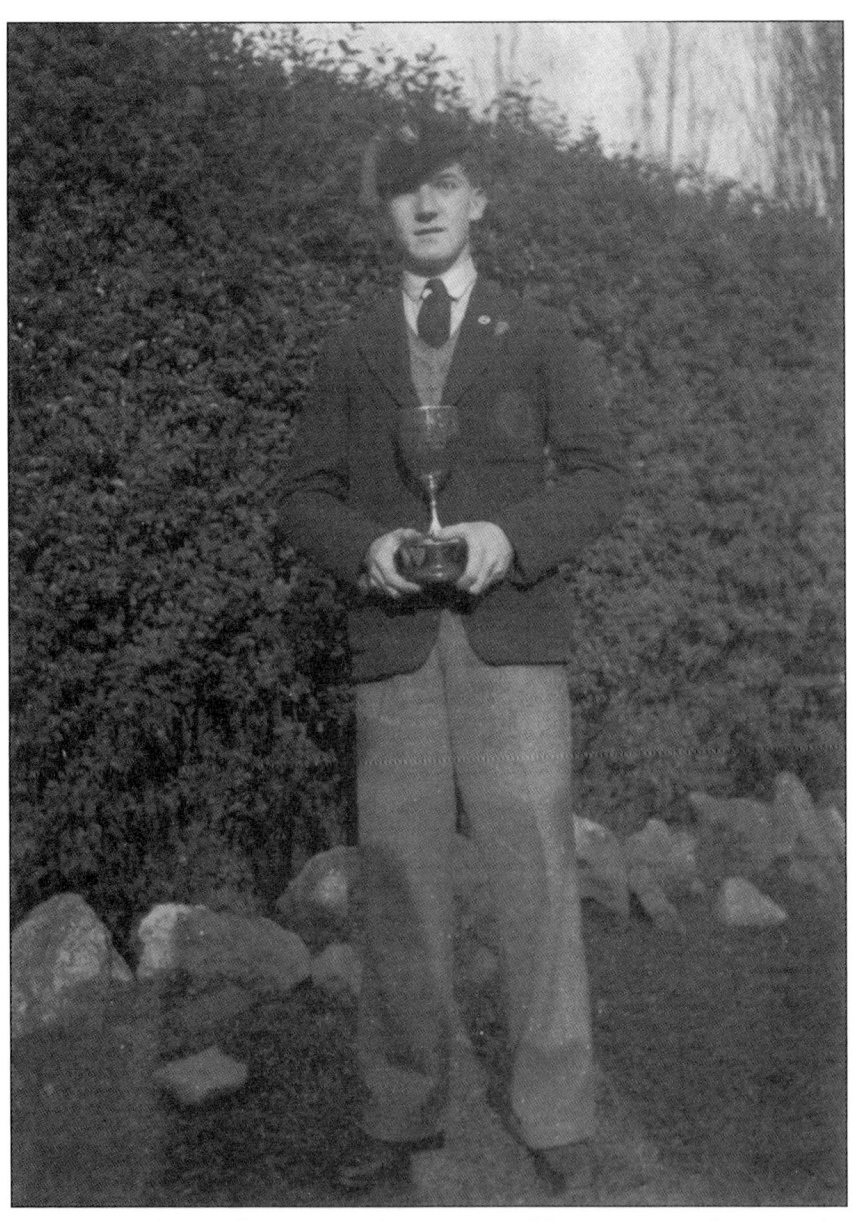

Summer 1943. The Senior Swimming Champion with cup. The jaunty angle of the School Captain's cap with tassel must have been appropriate at the time.

how it emerged that I might make my career in Medicine, as there was no family tradition in this profession but there was encouragement. My Chemistry master, the late Mr I.G. Jones thought that I should try for Cambridge. Mr Jones gave up all the mornings of his Easter vacation to coach me personally in Organic Chemistry so that I could take the first MB Examination at Cambridge externally in May. This I did and was successful, and was interviewed and then followed the offer of a place at St John's College, which I was delighted to accept. I cannot explain what followed but shortly afterwards I turned down the place at Cambridge in favour of going to Edinburgh. Perhaps I was influenced by the family's Scottish traditions and of course the Edinburgh Medical School had a distinguished reputation. I could have done both, gone to Cambridge first, then to Edinburgh for my clinical years. However, had I done this I would have finally graduated a year later (six years as an undergraduate instead of five years), and if this had happened I would not have met my wife. As will emerge later, my wife Jenny was to become an absolutely critical part of my life.

Although I was much in Yorkshire in subsequent years, I did not pay a full pilgrimage to Doncaster until 1993, fifty years after leaving school. I had a memorable escorted tour of the school, a visit to childhood homes, then to a country church where as School Captain I had shared in the dedication of a stained-glass window.

Then I made, nervously, a pre-arranged visit to the home of Mr Jones. He was now aged ninety-five, but he remembered only too well Richmond's bad behaviour and rejection of Cambridge. However we were able to have a very happy time together, sharing reminiscences. He knew how much I respected and owed to him and all was forgiven.

When I left Doncaster Grammar School, the Second World War was still at its height. On the night of the first day of the war, 3 September 1939, the air-raid sirens startled us all so we jumped out of bed and hurried into the depths of the cold cellar of the house where we were later to set up bunks. Father said, 'They will be over in their thousands,' but nothing was heard until the 'all clear'. Doncaster fortunately escaped much bombing but we had multiple nocturnal alerts because the town was in line with Hull, Sheffield and Manchester, a regular path for overhead bombers. Apart from this I think my main memories are Mr Chamberlain's declaration of war on the wireless on Sunday morning, 3 September, the sight of hundreds of sad and bedraggled army survivors of Dunkirk on Doncaster racecourse, the Battle of Britain, the North Africa and Italian campaigns and the invasion of Russia. The horror of the Holocaust did not emerge until later.

CHAPTER 3

Undergraduate Days at University of Edinburgh Medical School and First Hospital Appointment, 1943-8

T HE ENTRY TO Edinburgh Medical School was some 200, a quarter of which were girls. Being wartime, we were all young; a few were still aged sixteen but most were in the seventeen to nineteen bracket. There were a few boys from Accra in West Africa. There were large numbers of Edinburgh schoolboys still retaining their school loyalties and being a lone boy from South Yorkshire, I remember thinking that they were a bit of a 'shower'. However that feeling quickly abated and very many were soon to become my best friends and have remained so. Many students of course lived at home, others in halls of residence but some resided like me in 'digs'. I stayed for my whole five years in a top-floor flat in a tenement in the Marchmont area, looked after by a delightful old lady who had been widowed in the First World War. Apart from breakfast, I had every evening meal provided and on Saturdays and Sundays I also received lunch; the cost was £2 2s per week, rising to £2 5s.

Teaching of medicine in Edinburgh went back into the 1400s. Significant events followed with the Incorporation of Surgeons and Barber Surgeons being established in 1505. In the late 1500s a Town's College was founded and in 1681 the Royal College of Physicians of Edinburgh followed (see Chapter 9). Some of the physicians were much involved in

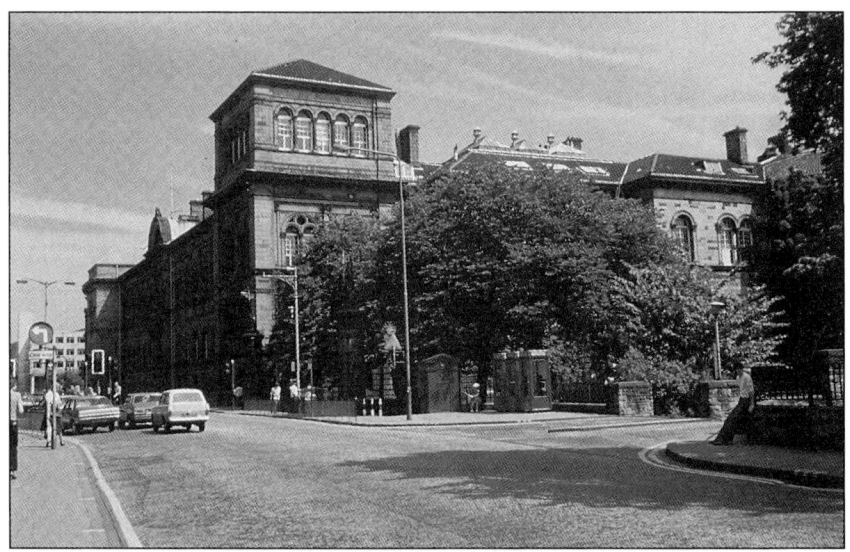

The Medical School in Teviot Place as it was in my time and as it is today. This houses the main departments of the preclinical and paraclinical subjects.

the creation of the Edinburgh Medical School but it is not widely known that it was the first to be established as a formal teaching Faculty in a University outside Oxford and Cambridge and this was in 1726. In those days in order to enter Oxford or Cambridge aspirants had to be members of the Church of England and so in the 1700s and 1800s students came in their droves from all parts of the United Kingdom, continental Europe and North America. Moreover in the 1700s Edinburgh was a particularly exciting place to be during 'The Enlightenment'.

The first professors had been mostly trained in Leiden, Holland and many of the early traditions had been inducted in them by the famous Professor Boerhaave. The first Professor of Medicine in the new University Medical School was John Rutherford, maternal grandfather of Walter

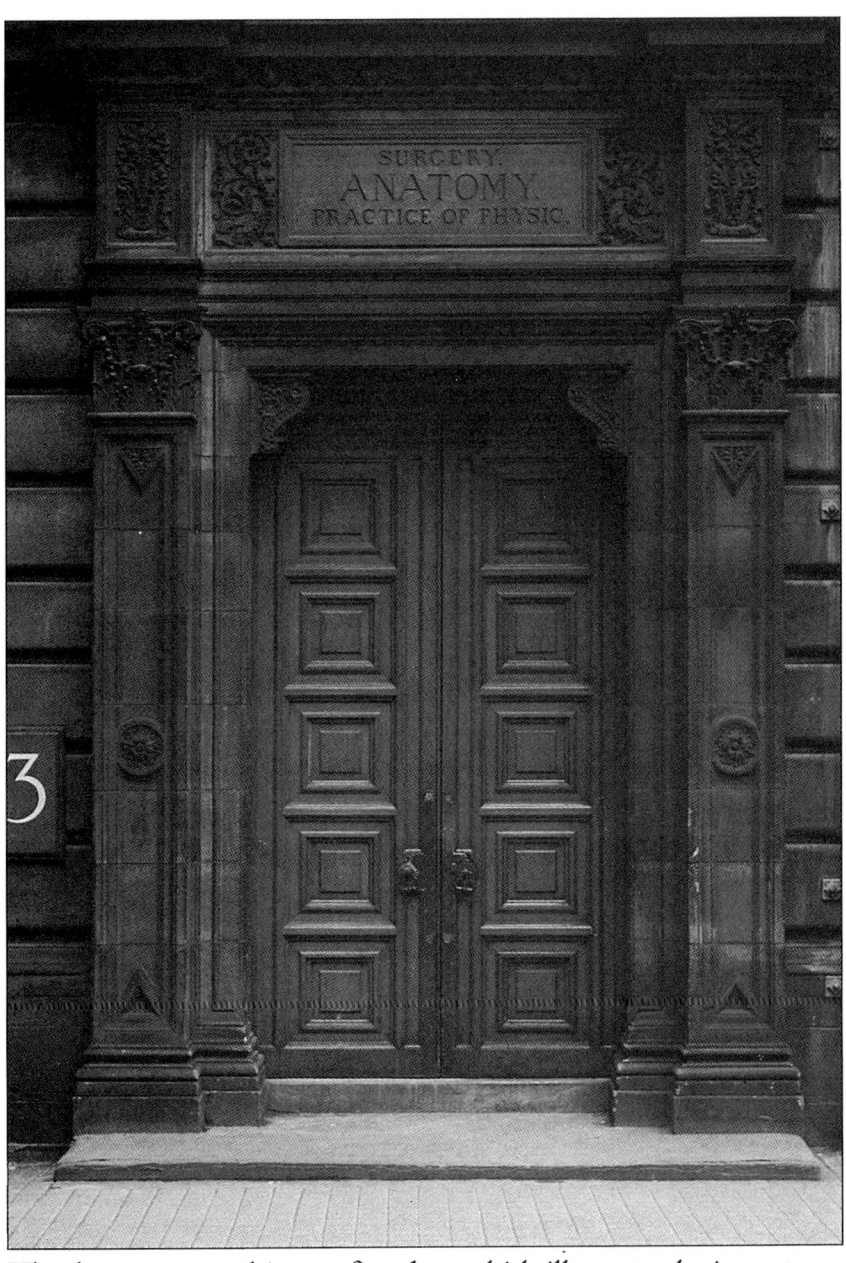

The door we entered in our first days which illustrates the importance
then of Anatomy compared with Surgery and the Practice of Physic.

Scott and it was he who started teaching clinical skills on living patients. There is a delightful recorded extract from Rutherford's first clinical lectures:

> The method I propose to pursue is to examine every patient before you, lest any circumstances should be overlooked. I shall conduct this by a plan which will be the most useful I can think of. I shall give you the history of this disease in general; second enquire into the cause of it; third give you my opinion how the disease is likely to terminate; lay down the indication of cure which will arise . . . If you find me mistaken I hope you will excuse me for the art of physic is not infallible . . . I shall make as accurate observations and as just conclusions as I can. I hope this will produce a good result and help to make you real physicians.

Clinical teaching was even more developed by the third Professor, William Cullen in the late 1700s. Indeed the founders of the first medical school in North America, in Philadelphia, received their medical training in Edinburgh in Cullen's time.

The early 1800s saw the evolution of Anatomy as an important discipline but sadly this period included the infamous 'body snatching'. Later, Surgery was to improve, particularly under Syme but aided by Lister's introduction of antisepsis and by the appearance of ether and then by the discovery of chloroform by the Professor of Midwifery, James Young Simpson.

In my time, the first year included Medical Chemistry, Physics, Zoology and Botany and in the second year there were three terms of Physiology. However both years were dominated by five terms of Anatomy when in pairs we dissected every part of the human body. The Professor of Anatomy was Professor Brash, who along with our Professor

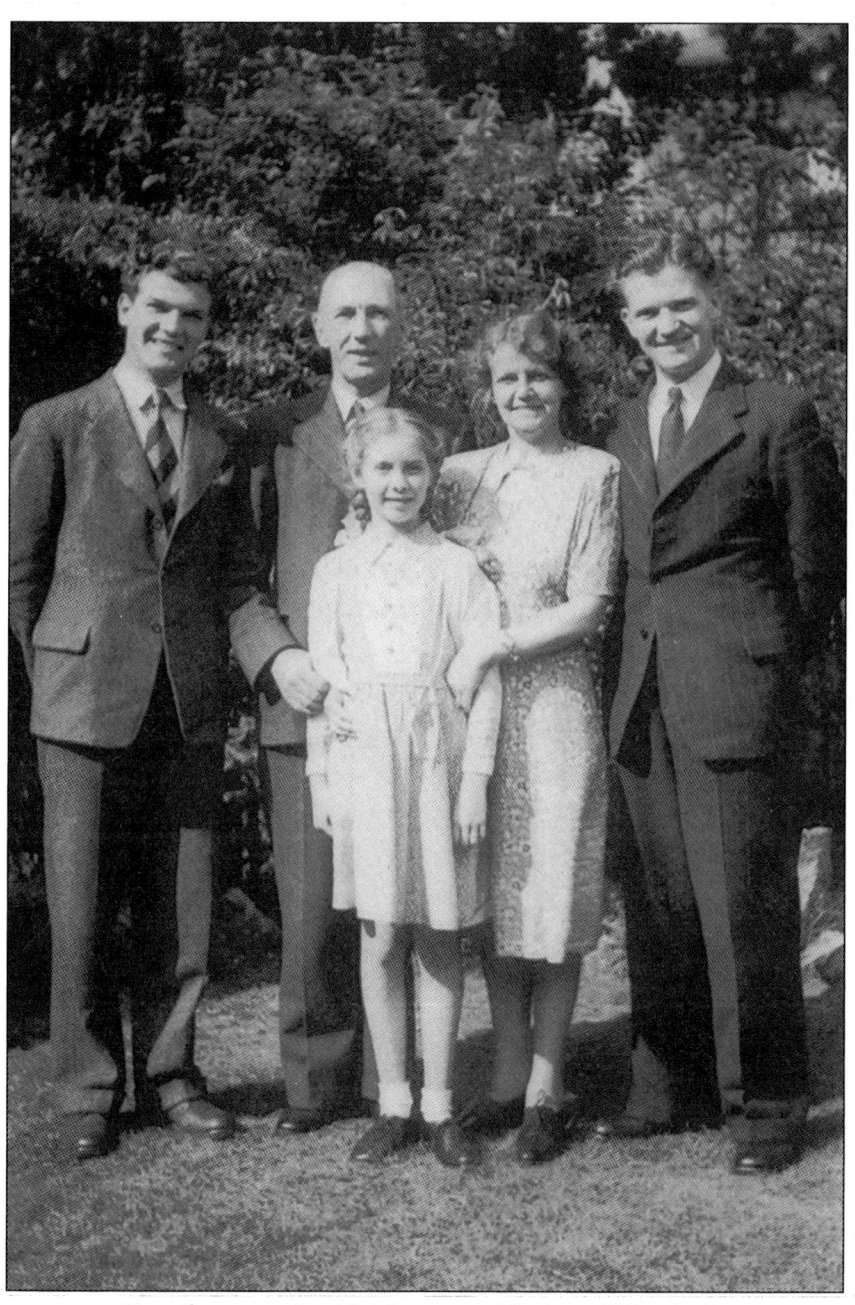

Family group in 1946, now with sister Elizabeth.

of Forensic Medicine and Dean, Sydney Smith, had had much to do with unravelling the Buck Ruxton murder case in the 1930s, a pioneering investigation. Our main dissecting room presence was the great Shetlander, Dr E.B. Jamieson. Indeed we were the last class to have him in his formal appointment, although he stayed around and continued to inspire succeeding classes of students.

Because of my English Higher School Certificate and Mr Jones, I was able to coast through my first year and concentrate on Anatomy. This led to my being awarded at the end of my second year the Cunningham Medal, so named after the famous Professor of Anatomy, Daniel Cunningham, father of the distinguished Second World War sailor, Admiral Cunningham. My head is still stuffed with all sorts of anatomical minutiae which I have never needed to use.

Being wartime, all the men had to belong compulsorily to the Senior Training Corps, the equivalent of the OTC. This lasted for our first two years and was quite a commitment. Every Wednesday afternoon we marshalled in High School Yards and after collecting our rifles were ordered by the Sergeant Major to get 'fell in three thick'. After inspection we would run at the double down the Cowgate and do three hours of manoeuvres near Holyrood Palace in King's Park on the slopes of Arthur's Seat. It was said that we would be expected to defend Daikeith in the event of invasion but of course fortunately this never happened. However once a term we were marched to Dalkeith to 'recce' the area and then returned to Edinburgh by coach with blistered feet.

Another memory I have of the STC was our having to take part in frequent parades along Princes Street such as 'Wings for Victory' and 'Salute the Soldier'. This would be in the summer of 1944. The parades would marshal in Waterloo Place, near St Andrew's House, and would include contingents from the Navy, Army, Air Force, Wrens, ATS and WAAFS and then us, and after us there would be Boy Scouts, Girl Guides, Boys Brigade and others. The parades would be about a mile long.

On one occasion, after setting off, our pipe band was about 100 yards ahead of the company that I was in and just behind us the Boy Scouts were blowing their bugles ten to the dozen. Passing the General Post Office, as we entered the east end of Princes Street we were all hopping and skipping to get into step, with our rifles at the slope. I remember very clearly hearing a voice from the pavement, 'Jings is thaes fellies dancin'?' (Goodness me are these fellows dancing?)!

The third year of the medical course was mainly Medicine and Surgery with collateral Pathology, Bacteriology and Therapeutics. Fourth year was mainly Obstetrics and Gynaecology, Psychiatry, Paediatrics and Public Health Medicine, together with so-called 'specials', ENT (ear, nose and throat), Ophthalmology and 'skins' (Dermatology). In the final year we returned mainly to Medicine and Surgery.

We all had to have delivered twelve babies in normal parturition but also had to have observed complicated childbirth during six weeks residence near the Simpson Maternity Pavilion of the Edinburgh Royal Infirmary. Many of us opted to do our normal midwifery based in Dublin either at the Coombe or the Rotunda Hospital. The childbirth experience was mostly in rather humble homes in the city and I recall occasions waiting for the baby to arrive with a picture of De Valera watching over me from one wall and the Sacred Heart from another. The group I

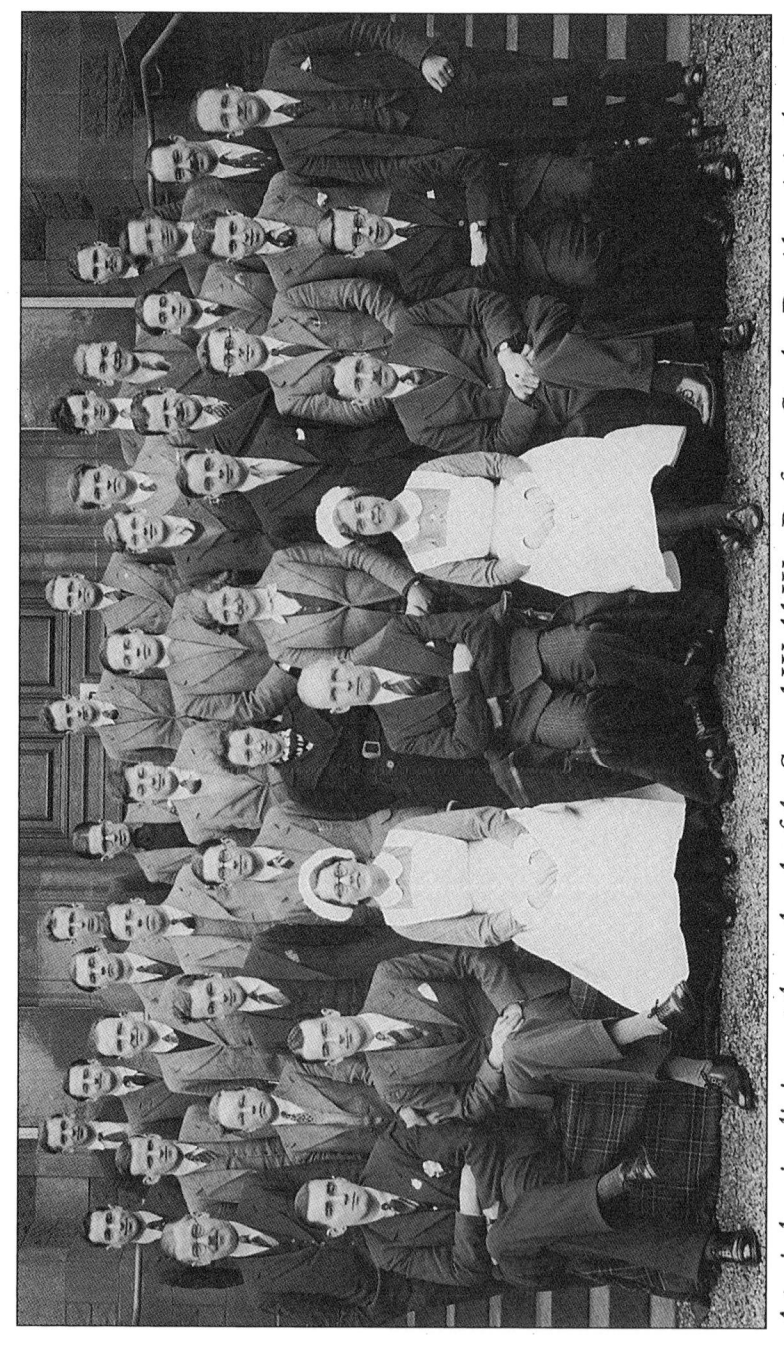

A typical senior clinique at the outbreak of the Second World War. Professor Stanley Davidson is in the centre with his ward sisters. His colleagues on the front row were all to become teachers of my class in 1945–8.

was with went out by boat from Glasgow and we did not get down to business for several days. We arrived on St Patrick's Day, which was followed by Holy Thursday and then Good Friday. But Saturday was committed also – everyone went to the races at Phoenix Park! One other memory is of the tavern next to the hospital known as the 'PPH'. We thought at first that this must mean 'post partum haemorrhage but were soon to learn that it was 'pub past hospital' and it seemed to be highly accessible even when closed.

Many skills were learned 'junioring' at nights in the hospital wards of the main teaching hospitals, particularly the Edinburgh Royal Infirmary. Perhaps more importantly we had long summer vacations and many of us worked in hospitals near our homes where, because of the war, young doctors were in short supply.

I once removed a small piece of steel from the thumb of the late Bruce Woodcock in the casualty department of Doncaster Royal Infirmary. This would be in the summer of 1946 or 1947. Fortunately it must have been a very minor event because he was then at the height of his career as British Heavyweight Boxing Champion.

The sporting interests continued. At first I concentrated on rugby, trying to stay in my favoured position as scrum half. Unfortunately the scrum half for Scotland, Angus Black, was also in my class and so I got to play for the first XV only when he was busy on a higher plain or unwell. One afternoon I was included when we played against a rather prestigious Royal Australian Air Force XV and we lost by a modest margin. The next day in 'Sporting Titbits' in the *Edinburgh Evening Dispatch* there was a brief note to the effect that 'Had A.W. Black been playing 'varsity might well have

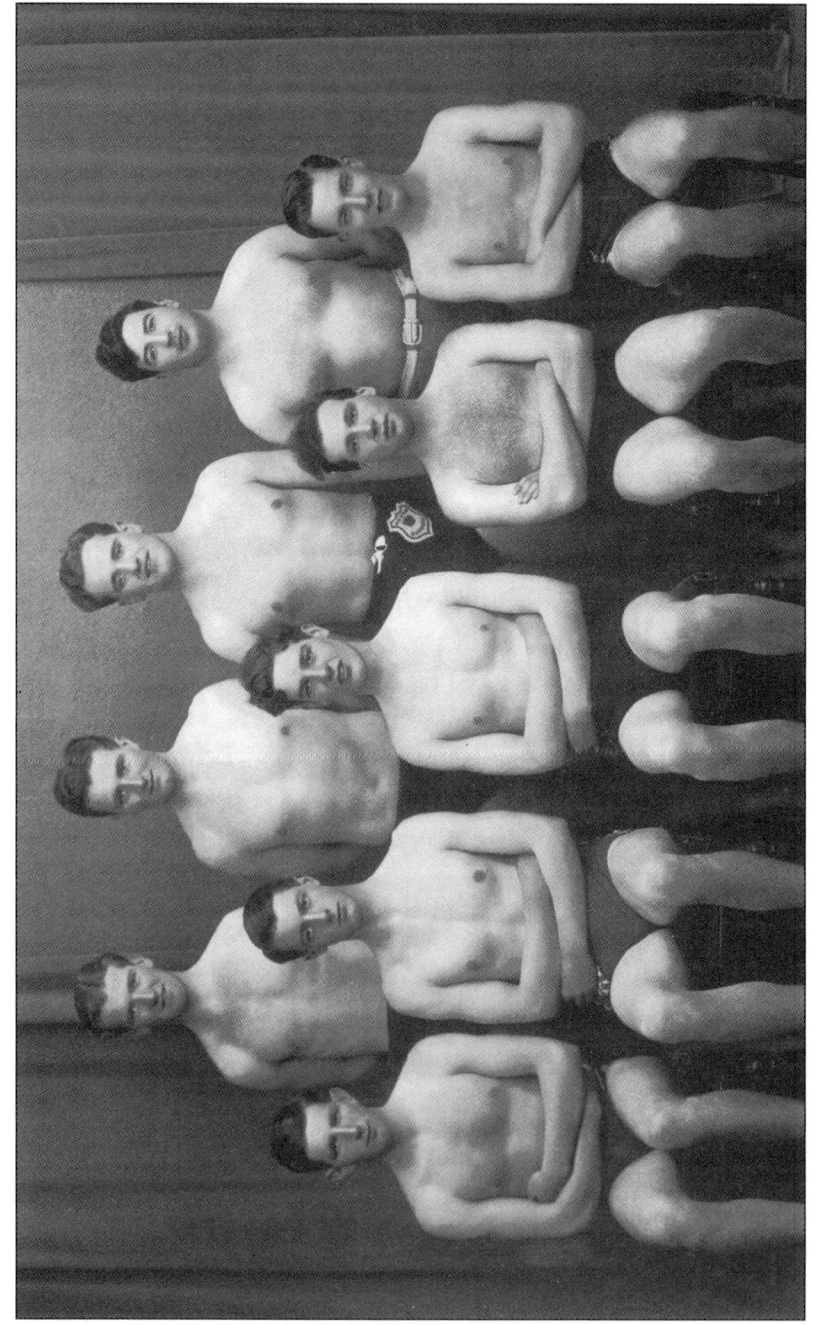

Swimming team year of obtaining 'blue' for diving. Author is first from left in back row.

won', but happily went on to say, 'Richmond played quite a plucky game.'

I felt it wise to return to swimming and was soon recruited into the university team. In 1947 we were the Inter-University Swimming Champions, winning every event. I had won the high board diving and the *Varsity Athletic News* had the nice entry, 'In J. Richmond we found a neat and reliable diver who got us honours in this event for the first time since P. Heatly graduated.' Peter Heatly of course went on to win the gold medal for diving in the Commonwealth Games. I did not get as far as this but was delighted with the award of a University 'Blue'. Now if I am standing three feet above the ground I feel dizzy!

Apart from these sporting interests, there were many other digressions. In the third year particularly, I recall many of us being bored by the Pathology lectures, immediately after lunch, important as they were. Lunch was usually a roast beef rissole and chips costing 10 old pence! Instead of dropping off to sleep a group would repair to Jack's Billiard Saloon nearby and we soon became quite expert at billiards and snooker. This perhaps explains why my sons were so puzzled by my knowing where the coloured balls were in snooker contests, when we still had black and white tele-vision. We also had a good billiard room in the University Men's Union. I enjoyed being on the Union Committee of Management in the Final Year. The Committee included several members of staff but also encouraged much mixing with other students and attendance at the regular jolly Saturday evening dances – the 'Union Palais'.

I have to reflect again on the many outstanding teachers I was exposed to in the Edinburgh Medical School and at that time most of the bedside clinical teaching was done by the

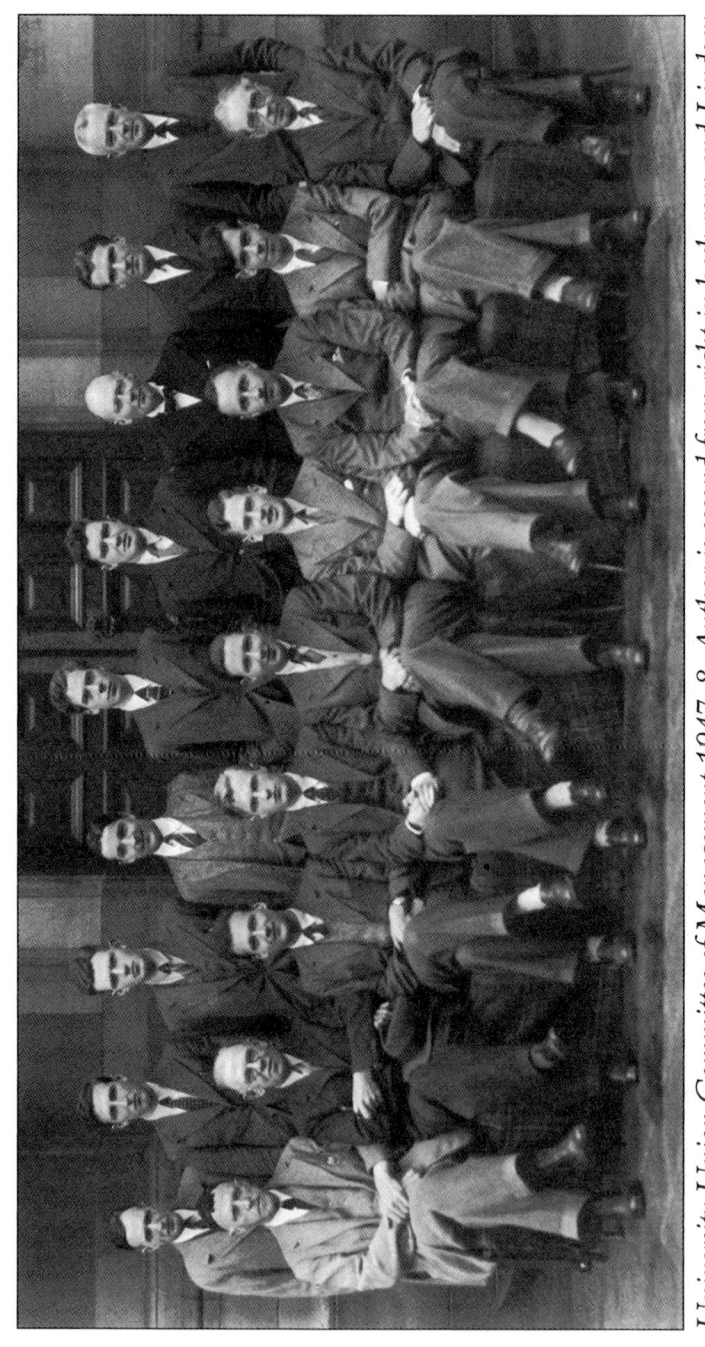

University Union Committee of Management 1947-8. Author is second from right in back row and Lindsay Davidson, his opposite number in the Deaconess Hospital, is fourth from right. Another long-standing friend, Douglas Bell was President and is seated fifth from right in the front row. Dr E.B. Jamieson and Professor Brash are first and second from the left on the front row.

most senior. My class and near contemporaries had the great Stanley Davidson, Derrick Dunlop, Rae Gilchrist, James Learmouth, David Henderson and many others all prepared to give endless time to their clinical work and their teaching. Stanley Davidson used to say that if you took a good history from a patient and then did a careful examination, the rest might not be too difficult or too expensive. This is still true.

I passed the Final Professional Examination with Distinction and we graduated on 12 July 1948 one week after the inception of the National Health Service. I do not think that many of us had much idea what the National Health Service meant, or was going to mean.

A few other things happened in 1948. For example, cortisone was introduced and vitamin B12, the treatment for pernicious anaemia was isolated from liver. We already had sulphonamides and following penicillin, other anti-biotics were beginning to emerge. We also had digitalis and barbiturates and morphine and aspirin, but the range of medicines was fairly limited.

In Edinburgh at that time one registered with the General Medical Council on graduation and pre-registration House Officer jobs in hospital had not become obligatory. Most of us would join the MDDUS, the Medical and Dental Defence Union of Scotland, for which the annual subscription was then one guinea (£1 1s). House Officer appointments lasted for six months and began in October and April. If I remember correctly, I believe that in 1948 we were only permitted to do one job before being called up for eighteen months (later two years) military service, but there were some grounds for deferment and of course exclusion because of ill health. Many of my class went into hospitals all over the country and some for a time went straight into

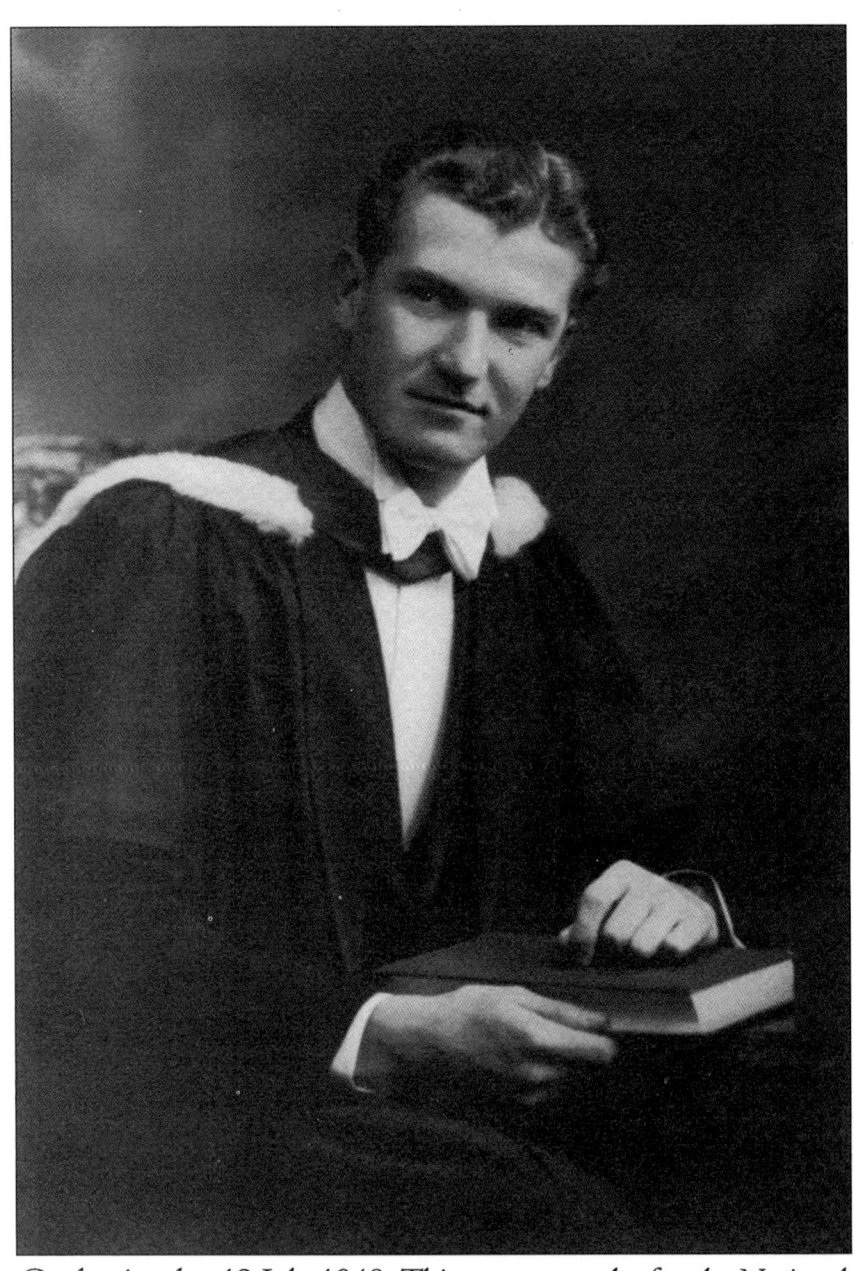

Graduation day 12 July 1948. This was one week after the National Health Service started on 5 July.

general practice. I opted to do a House Officer job in Edinburgh in a small hospital sharing duties with a classmate, Lindsay Davidson.

I filled in part of the August and September months by doing a few weeks in a locum appointment in Baguley Sanatorium in Cheshire near Manchester. This was a large hospital and it was a revelation indeed to see so many patients with active tuberculosis, mostly in the younger age groups, and to experience the level of mortality. At that time there were no curative medicines and the treatment involved bed rest, with rest of the affected lung by pneumothorax (air in the pleural space), pneumoperitoneum (air in the abdomen), phrenic nerve crush in the neck to paralyse the diaphragm and sometimes mutilating surgery termed thoracoplasty when ribs were removed. Apart from assisting at thoracoplasties I had to undertake the other procedures and the many patients with air in their body spaces had to receive refills every week.

The House Officer job began on 1 October in the Deaconess Hospital, Edinburgh. This was a remarkable period and perhaps in retrospect a most unusual experience. The hospital had been associated with the Church of Scotland but was now embraced by the NHS. Lindsay Davidson and I were of course resident and we looked after about 120 acute hospital beds which included adult medical and surgical wards, a children's ward and a number of beds set aside for gynaecology and ENT patients. There was a casualty department which could be quite busy. The two of us did three months predominantly on the medical side and three months on the surgical side. Our consultant staff to whom we were responsible were all primarily based in the Edinburgh Royal Infirmary, but were all readily available if

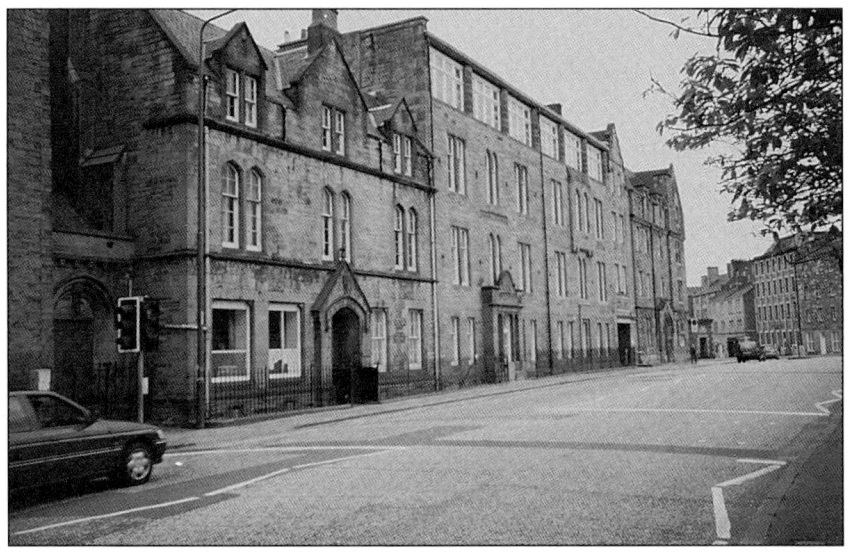

Deaconess Hospital, Edinburgh, now Lothian Health Board offices. This was where I held my first House Officer appointment, October 1948 to March 1949.

called upon. They all did regular ward rounds and there were several operating sessions each week. At that time no undergraduate students were being taught in the hospital which meant that they could not share some of the tasks. A few young doctors leaving the Services attended the hospital primarily as observers but they did stand in for us and support us in times of pressure. The two House Officers therefore carried considerable responsibility. They had to do minor surgery and reduce simple fractures in the casualty department, where they might also have to give simple anaesthetics. We also gave the anaesthetics to children in tonsil operations. We worked late into the night counting blood cells, staining blood films and bone marrow smears, and testing urine samples. Major investigations were done at the Infirmary. None of this would have been possible without the help, advice, assistance and even instruction by the outstanding ward sisters and staff nurses. Throughout my entire professional life the nursing profession has been an essential partner.

Looking back, one particular medical problem was beginning to emerge which I do not recall being taught on when I was a medical student, and that was myocardial infarction (coronary thrombosis). Dr Ian Hill (later Professor of Medicine in Dundee), was very interested in cardiology and at that time was pioneering the further development of electrocardiography. He was our senior physician.

My pay for the first month was £4 1s 6d later adjusted to the new NHS scales. We did of course have free board and lodging but the salary did not matter because we were seldom able to get out of the hospital to spend it. I will however recall two outings.

One evening my opposite number held the fort while I went out to the Royal Infirmary to see some old pals. I did not realise that every time my glass of beer was half empty it was being filled up and the result was that around midnight I had to be returned to the Deaconess Hospital in the Dalkeith ambulance. The Night Sister was not very pleased with me.

The other outing also upset the Night Sister. In those days peptic ulcer, particularly duodenal ulcer, was common and often intractable. Many patients ended up having gastric surgery and often had a month of intensive medical treatment in hospital before surgery was decided upon. One patient was a general practitioner but I seem to remember that he had disguised the fact that he was a young doctor and had served in RAF aircrew during the war. In any case he was rather an unusual chap.

After a few days of milk and alkali, milk puddings and steamed fish he said, 'Richmond, I cannot stand this any longer'. I had to say, 'I am not at all surprised but what am I to do?' 'Well,' he said, 'Chico Marx is on at the Empire Theatre and I would love to go.' To cut a long story short my colleague again held the fort while my doctor patient and I slipped out through the boiler house, because I, of course, had to take him. We had a grand evening but Sister caught us soon after returning through the boiler house. However there were no harsh words because she was so relieved to find her missing patient alive and well. I think that the patient's symptoms were much better next day.

At a medical examination at the Cowglen Military Hospital in Glasgow early in 1949, I was passed fit for military service. My time at the Deaconess Hospital ended on 31 March and I was called into the Royal Army Medical Corps two weeks later. I was still only twenty-two years old but I think Colonel Keyes was only twenty-two when he led the raid on Rommel's headquarters and Guy Gibson was only twenty-four when he led 'the Dambusters'!

CHAPTER 4

Military Service in Africa, 1949-50

AFTER SIX WEEKS induction at Crookham near Aldershot and at Millbank in London our first postings began. Many were assigned to the United Kingdom. I volunteered to go to the Middle East and a most maturing experience followed.

Those going to the Middle East and Far East went out on the troopship SS *Dunera*, later to be named the SS *Uganda*. Six of us were crammed into a cabin meant for three. We rounded Cape St Vincent at Gibraltar to our first stop at Port Said. One of our six spent most of his time sitting on his bunk blowing a chanter (the musical part of bagpipes), and he nearly ended up going through the porthole into the Mediterranean. Quite fortuitously the piper and I were to become close collaborators in research in the 1960s.

We arrived at Port Said in the dark and anchored offshore. Almost immediately we were surrounded by scores of little rowing boats known as 'bum boats', whose occupants were selling their wares up and down ropes to the troops hanging over the side or through portholes. On board was a battalion of the Argyll and Sutherland Highlanders en route to Hong Kong. I happened to look out of my porthole to see a kilted Highlander standing up on the ship's rail. At the same time one of his mates from a porthole low down shouted up to him, 'Pee on them, Jock', and he did, much to the consternation of the visitors.

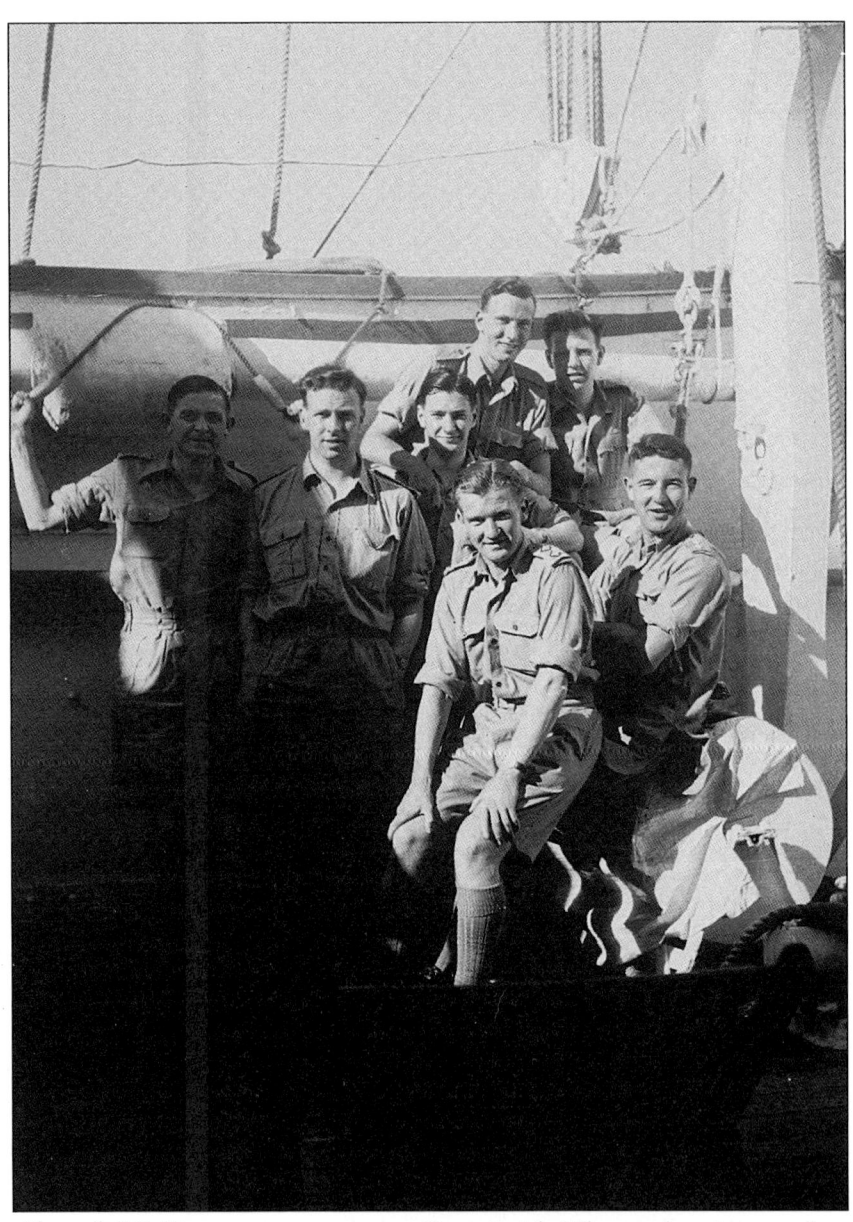

Aboard SS Dunera *en route to Port Said. The author is seated at front and Angus Stuart (the chanter player), a research colleague in the 1960s, is immediately behind.*

Next morning before disembarking a 'Gilligilli' man (spelling uncertain), came on board and as part of his act, produced scores of little chickens from under his white gown. Then after getting off the boat, we were greeted by small boys, 'Hello Mr Churchill', 'Hello Harry Lauder', 'You like meet my sister?' But we were soon on our way to the transit camp down the west side of the Suez Canal.

After two weeks I was posted to the Military Mission in Ethiopia to relieve its Medical Officer for two months, I think selected because of the brief but very varied experience in the Deaconess Hospital. I was a little nervous, not having travelled overseas before and because of continuing local unrest after the Palestine conflict, I was not allowed to travel in uniform. The train to Cairo left from Ismailia where the station was swarming with people. When the train came in, many passengers were hanging on the outside, but I managed to get on board. After walking up and down, I eventually found a compartment full of packing cases with a stocky gentleman sitting in one corner. There was a little sitting space in another corner and I asked in slow English did he mind if I joined him. 'Not at all, lad, come in. I'm Mr "So and so" from Bayswater, travelling for Burberry's, just back from China.' Mr 'So and so' was a good companion and we had dinner together that evening at the famous restaurant in Cairo, Groppi's, before I caught my plane.

The flight to Ethiopia was in a noisy Dakota, stopping first at Jeddah, which now has one of the most sophisticated airports in the world, but in 1949 the airport was like a small broken-down English cricket pavilion. From the air one could see overland trails to Mecca. Then on to Asmara in Eritrea, and over the mountains to Addis Ababa.

I did not have much opportunity to travel widely in

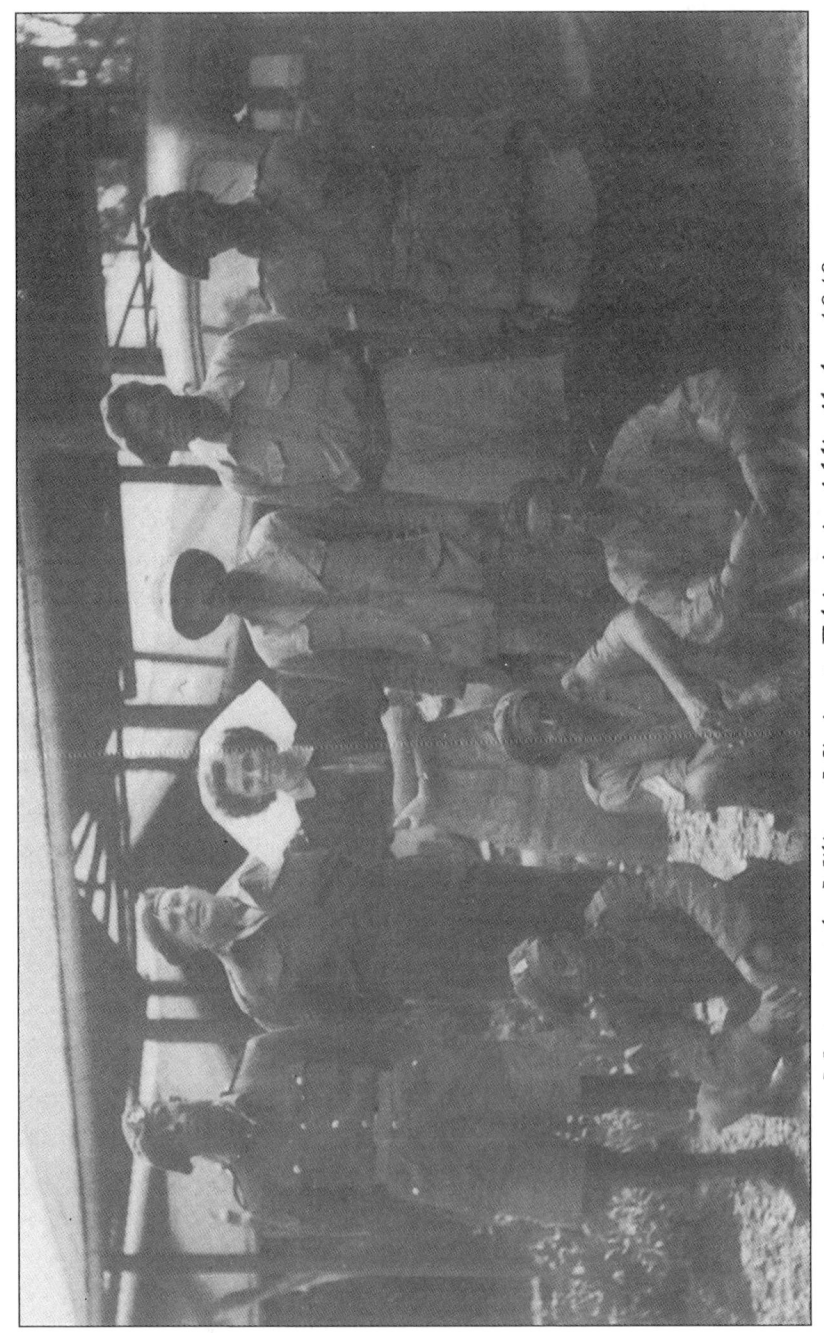

My team at the Military Mission to Ethiopia in Addis Ababa, 1949.

Ethiopia. The capital had some fine buildings such as Haile Selassie's Palace (and Haile Selassie was in residence at the time), and the Koptik Church. The Italians had left behind a railway station and an opera house but Via Mussolini had become Via Churchill.

I often look back on those few weeks with alarm. The Military Mission comprised a Major General, senior officers and many NCOs whose purpose seemed to be to train the Imperial Ethiopian Army. I was the only British doctor in the country, although there were a few Scandinavian doctors and also a small Russian hospital, where I was not welcome. There was also quite a large Russian legation. I wonder how I would have handled a serious medical problem because Nairobi was 400 miles away and British military hospitals in Egypt a good deal further. Fortunately there were no disasters. I did however have two rather challenging surgical procedures on very large dogs, each of which required anaesthesia. The first dog had buckled its big tail rather badly, and the owners asked me if it could be corrected. All I could do was to perform an amputation. The second dog had jumped over a barbed-wire fence, torn the scrotum and had a testis hanging out. Again, fortunately, all was well. Interestingly, reflecting on the Russian presence in 1949, much of that 'Horn of Africa' later became Marxist.

I flew to Nairobi on another noisy Dakota of Ethiopian Airlines with the Lion of Judah painted on the tail and crewed by Trans World Airlines. There were few passengers and I was sitting at the back, minding my own business, when I was aware above the noise of someone shouting in my ear, 'We are crossing the equator right now and that is Mount Kenya on the left there.' As I turned round the lovely air hostess was kneeling beside me and unfortunately the top of her dress had fallen rather far forward. Although this may sound indelicate I am afraid that I was temporarily distracted from the scenery that I was supposed to admire!

The time at the military hospital at Mackinnon Road between Voi and Mombasa was most educational and rewarding. There were several very good medical officers and Queen Alexandra nursing sisters. We had a commanding officer and supervisory physician. My own job was to do three large sick parades in surrounding camps each morning and also to be in charge of a medical ward. Some Swahili had to be mastered fairly quickly for the sick parades. 'Nahara' (diarrhoea) was common and treated from the so-called MI Rooms with 'Mist. kaolin sed'. 'Nahara damu', diarrhoea with blood, usually meant dysentery, and admission to the hospital. When the sick Askaris got to know how I handled this, I one day caught a group queuing up to see me with their obligatory stool samples and some were pricking their finger to add some 'damu'! My memory of Swahili may not be quite the same as in present-day dictionaries.

A major event was a large outbreak of typhoid fever, despite all the troops having received TAB vaccination. The mortality was rising to high levels when fortunately the new and effective antibiotic, chloramphenicol, became available and helped to stop the epidemic.

There were one or two interesting trips to Nairobi and Mombasa, and one to Moshi to view the snow-capped Mount Kilimanjaro. On all these journeys wild animals of all kinds were numerous. One duty which I had to undertake personally was to travel north once a month to the River Tsavo to inspect the source of our water supply. There was plenty of wild life in that area and the book, *The*

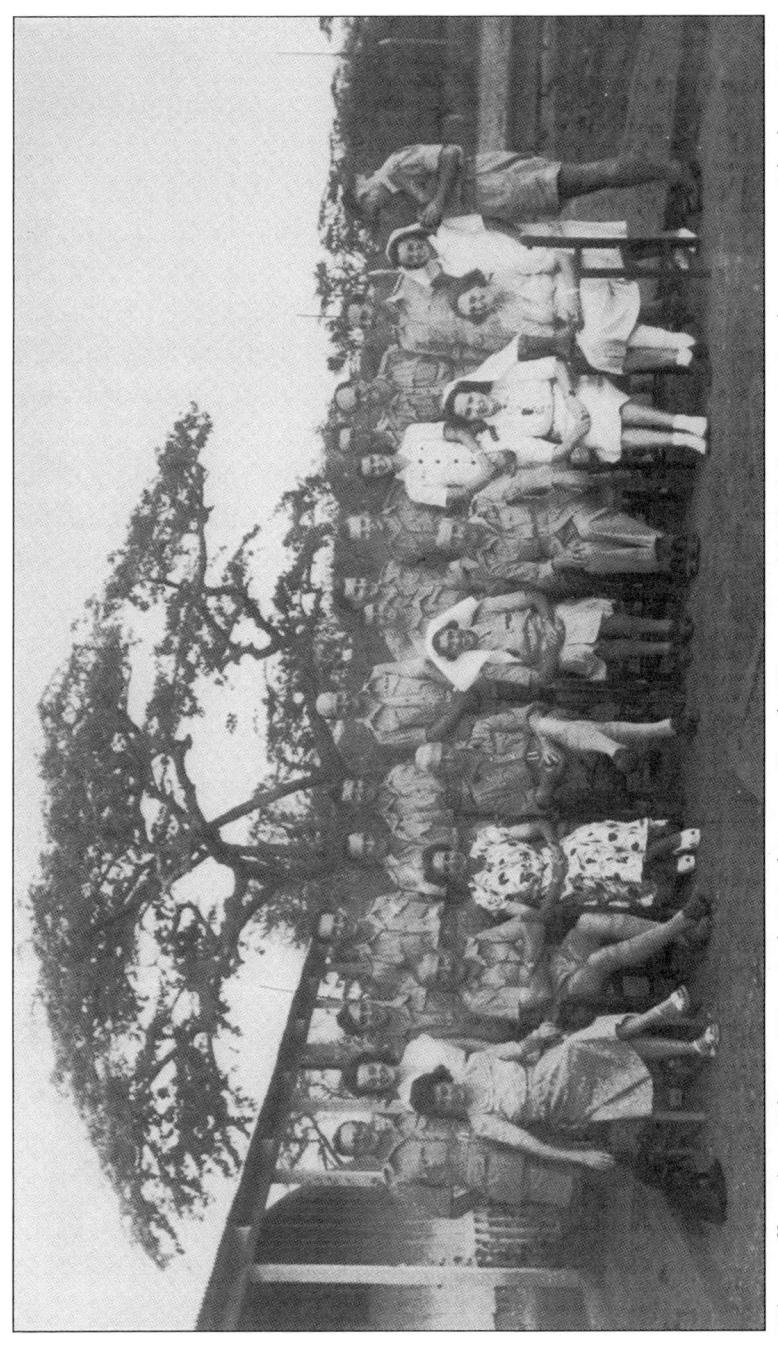

The staff at the Military Hospital, Mackinnon Road, Kenya in 1949. Matron is in the centre with the visiting Director of Medical Services and Assistant Director on either side. The author is sixth from the left in the back row.

Man Eaters of Tsavo, was based on some lion attacks on the early railway workers.

Christmas was approaching and I was looking forward to having a role in the pantomime. Then out of the blue, I was posted to be the Medical Officer to the 1st Nyasaland Battalion of the King's African Rifles, based in Lusaka, Northern Rhodesia. Again this was to be another great part of life's tapestry. The King's African Rifles were extensively involved in the Second World War, but were now reduced to a few security battalions in Africa. Idi Amin was later to be a Sergeant Major in the Uganda battalion.

My duties were less onerous than in Mackinnon Road, but nonetheless enhanced my further training. The British Officers and NCOs and their families presented few problems, and the same was true of the Africans. I did a sick parade at 06.30 hours every morning and because of the general fitness of the troops (and their families), much of

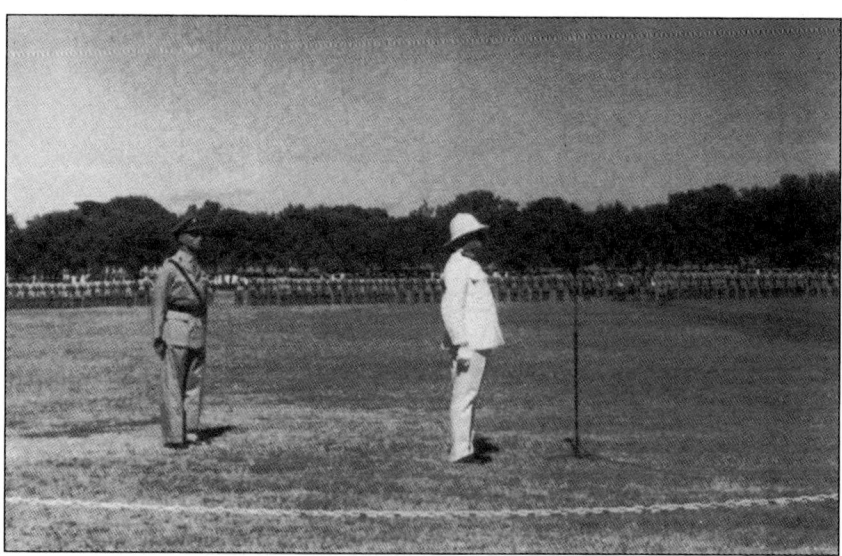

1st (Ny) Bn King's African Rifles.

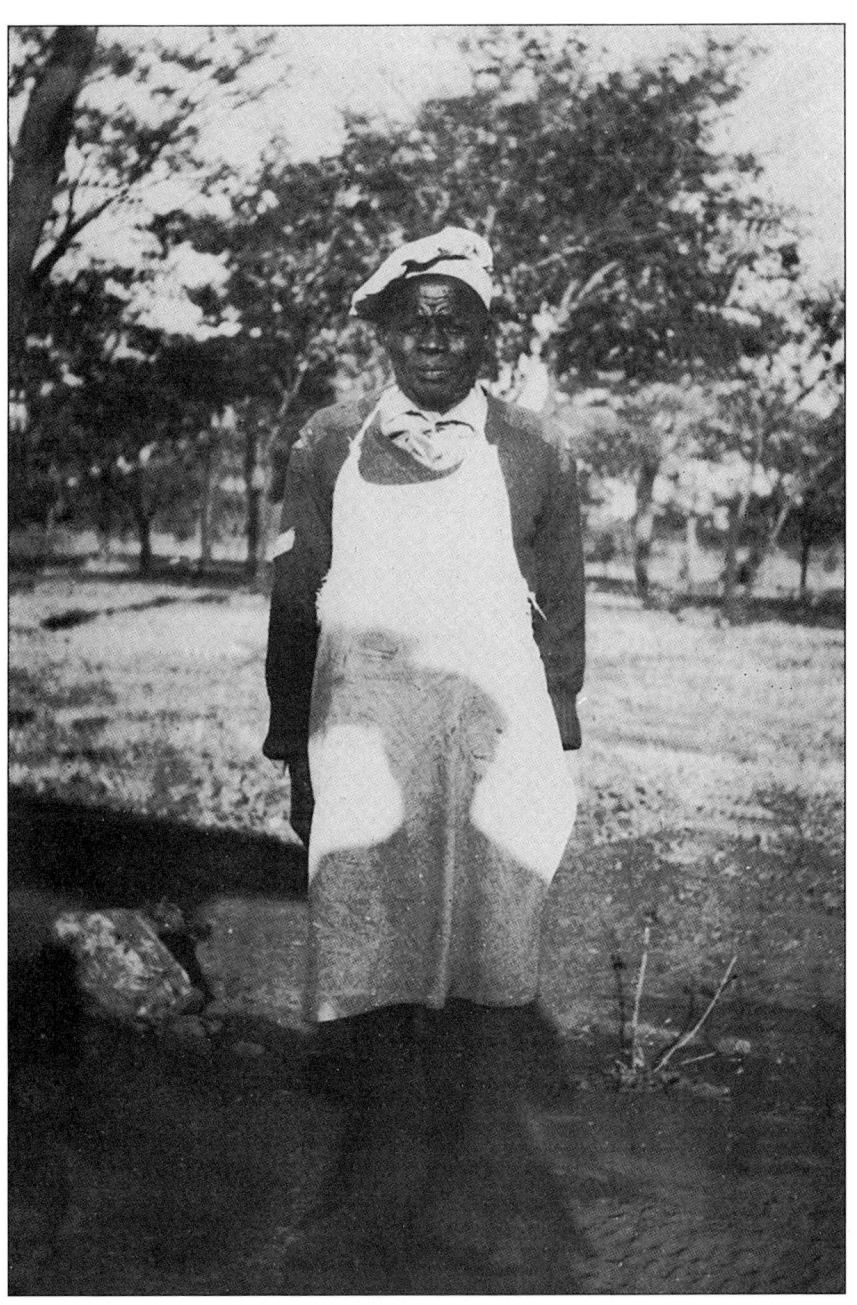

Corporal Jonathan.

the day's work could be achieved by breakfast time or soon after. I had a little sick bay of my own, with a few beds for minor illness and there were very good if small European and African hospitals in Lusaka which gave support. Indeed I often assisted at operations in the European hospital in the mornings. There were few doctors in Lusaka and most in Northern Rhodesia at that time were based in the copper belt in the north.

My greatest fan was the battalion cook, Corporal Jonathan. Goodness knows how old he was. He wore a medal dated 1908 which was from one of the Mad Mullah's uprisings in Somalia, but I never liked to ask him if it had really been awarded to him.

Among Jonathan's particular requests was that I would deliver his granddaughter of his first great-grandchild in my little hospital. This of course occurred early one morning without difficulty and I went back to see her an hour or two later only to find that she had gone to the market with the baby on her back. Jonathan was delighted and told me that that afternoon the family had made 'Merry Christmas from 2 p.m. to 4 p.m.'.

I had my first involvement with witchcraft. The sergeant in the Officers' Mess occasionally helped me with some of the ailments that appeared to be non-organic, with all sorts of strange herbal remedies. However the event that sticks in my memory most strongly related to a particular soldier, Chibaya. He had learned that for some reason the elders of his tribe in Nyasaland had put a spell on his beer. Gradually he began to fade away and in the little sick bay he lay in bed with face turned to the wall awaiting death. With some difficulty I persuaded the Commanding Officer to let my dying patient return to Nyasaland on one of the convoys so that Chibaya could make peace with the elders and have the spell lifted. He returned fully restored a month or so later.

Some months into my time in Lusaka there followed a most critical event. I was the bar member in the Officers' Mess and one day the Commanding Officer intimated that he would like to have a cocktail party on the Saturday evening. Apart from the officers and their wives, we would be having some guests from Government and the local hospitals and the police. He requested that I would prepare his favourite cocktail, something that I had never heard of: a 'White Lady'. With difficulty I discovered that it was gin and Cointreau and lemon squash, but no one seemed to know if it was 1:2:3, or 2:1:3 or whatever.

I spent the Saturday afternoon finding out and by 4 o'clock I was 'legless'. However after an hour or so in bed, I was feeling normal again and able to attend the cocktail party. Then as usually happened on a Saturday evening, a fair number of us chose to go to the weekly dinner dance at the Country Club.

I had a girlfriend who had a wobbly old car and she and I went to the Club with another officer and his wife in the back seat. I was still feeling my normal self, but the first strange happening was that a police officer slipped on the dance floor and dislocated his shoulder. I made the diagnosis with unjustified confidence and then reduced the dislocation with Kocher's manoeuvre, something that I had never done before, and have not done since. However, although my patient did look a little pale, all was well.

Then on the way home, I was driving and as we rounded the corner outside Government House the car skidded, I think on sand, and I was thrown out onto the road; the car fell across me. If I had been smoking I would not have survived because I was soaked in petrol. Fortunately my passengers were unharmed. However it took half an hour or so to get help to lift the car from me, and because I was having trouble with sensation and movement in my legs I was taken into the local hospital. Happily there was no serious injury, and on recovery one of my mates came to collect me at the hospital in my own little army 'buggy', so that I could drive back to the barracks and restore my confidence. However the first thing that I had to do was go to the bank.

Everyone in the small European community in Lusaka knew that the army doctor had made a fool of himself and the next person in the bank queue was a most attractive young lady whom I had met briefly once before. Her greeting was, 'You should take more water with it next time.' This was Jenny aged twenty, who was later to become a marvellous wife, companion, and consort. I was to discover that her parents also came from the west of Scotland where she had been born, but she had been brought up in Hertfordshire to where her father had moved his farming in the early 1930s. She had been preceded in Africa by an older sister, and Jenny had gone out some two years later staying for one year in Johannesburg and working with the Anglo-American Company and then moving to Lusaka, to friends, where she was to be in government service.

Shortly our friendship was to be interrupted because with an infantry officer and a transport officer, I was sent off into the south-west of Northern Rhodesia to assist in the recruitment of 200 men for the Northern Rhodesia Regiment, currently in Tanganyika. Each officer had a 15 cwt truck with driver and batman, and we were followed by 16 three-ton trucks for the recruits. We went south down the

Livingstone Road to Chomo and then westwards to Namwala, an area that had not been recruited for some time.

I do not know how the 'bush telegraph' functioned, but the villages on our journey seemed to know that we were coming and the local Chief had arranged a congregation of young men. Charlie Matthews, the infantry officer, would give a short address, the Chief would advise the men not to join us too light heartedly because they would be away for three years and then some would rise and go and collect a few belongings. After I had made a superficial medical examination, off we would go.

We three officers slept in the open under mosquito nets beside an enormous fire. Although we did not see any lions, we could certainly hear them roaring not too far away. We fed mainly on guinea fowl, spur-wing geese, snub-nose duck and little sucking pigs. As we went on, accumulating men, some large animal such as a kudu or a wildebeest had to be shot most days, usually by Charlie. We had brought a lot of provisions with us, which I remember included Booth's gin. We also had a battery radio with fairly clear reception.

By Namwala we had a large number of recruits and so twelve trucks were sent back to Lusaka. We went on to Sesheke on the Zambesi expecting to get along the north side of the river to return to base. Here we met the Paramount Chief in all his splendid robes, and he was anxious that we should meet his son. The son appeared out of a mud hut, in Savile Row suit and hat, an Oxford graduate!

Unfortunately we could not get along the north side of the river and had to cross cautiously on pontoons into the Caprivi Strip and from there eastwards. We arrived at the Victoria Falls on the night of a full moon to witness the

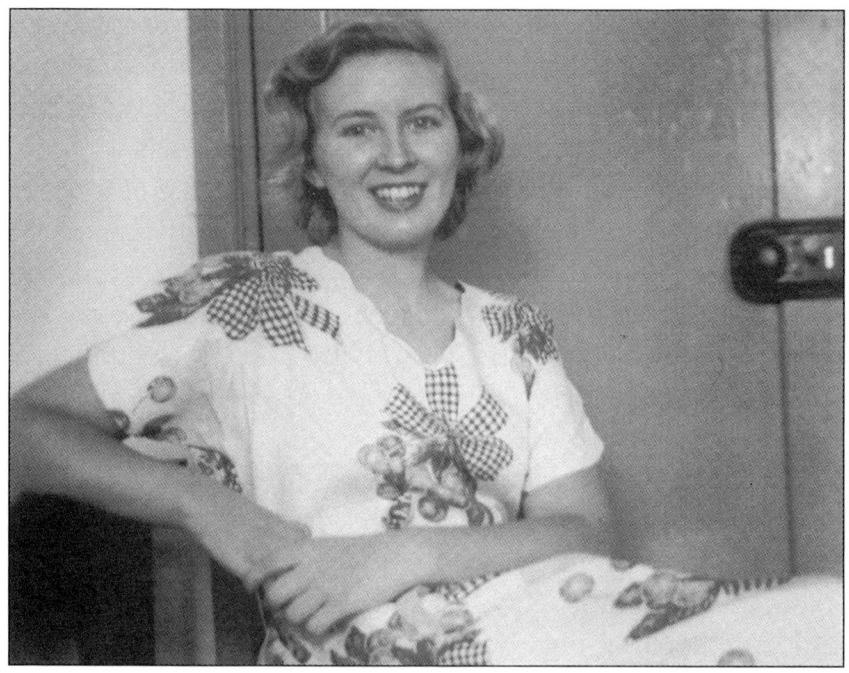

Jenny at the end of my time in Lusaka.

famous lunar rainbow in the spray. Then back to Lusaka into the embrace of my new lady.

I had given Charlie Matthews a £5 float when we set off and to my astonishment I got £4 change after our month's absence. We had had to buy only a few eggs and chickens. I, in addition, had had my army stipend doubled with one month's 'hard living allowance'! I also reflect on how we had all survived the water supply, because all we could do was to boil large volumes every day from rivers and small lakes.

Soon I was on my way home to the UK via a two-month camp in Southern Rhodesia where we had a busy spell of manoeuvres with troops from Kenya and Nyasaland but mainly Southern Rhodesia Territorials. It was yet another new experience.

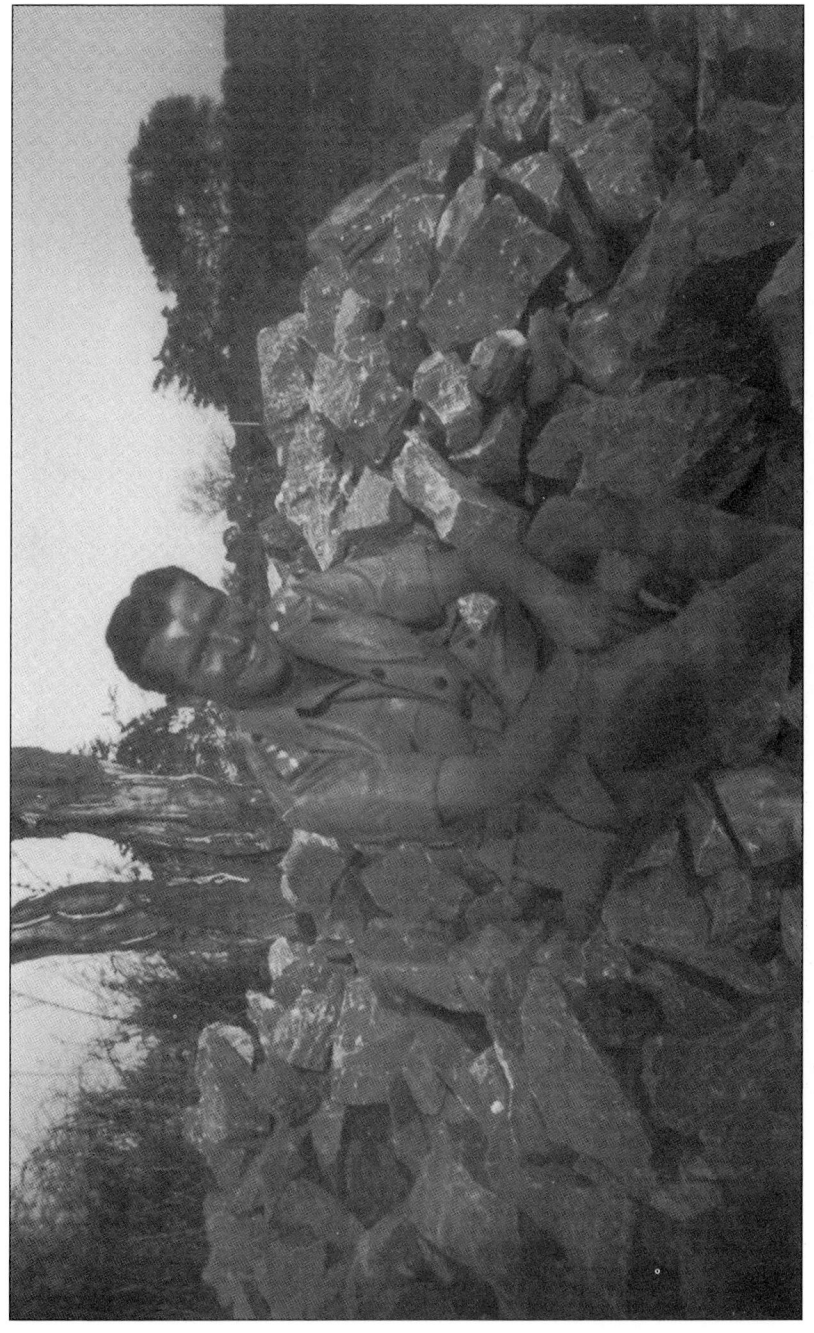

The author on last evening in Lusaka, 1950. Not exactly 'on the rocks'.

Bwana Love Doctor

T. B. "Coy"
1 K.A.R.
P.O. Box. 131.
Lusaka N.R.
28/8/50

1 K.A.R.
Enkomo Camp.
South Rhodesia

Dear Sir,

Many Many thanks Many Many thanks. Since I Born I never See Such a Doctor like yourself, My wife is return back from African Hospital date 24/8/50, Myself I was not believe that I will See my wife any more, But, by will of God I see my wife,

Sir, Very Very happy & Jamping like Air plain amsure, I trust now that you Said truth, for Sickness of my wife, I also I thanks to African Hosp. Doctor to give a good treatment to my wife, to Save Her in Danger Way, I hope that you Both are Very well in Camp their, no more to Say

Your humble & obedient Servant

ZBK13481. Cpl G. Jonathan. K. aphiri

Corporal Jonathan's letter to me in Southern Rhodesia.
'Both' in the penultimate line of the letter is because my
successor as MO had now arrived.

One nice event was to receive a letter from Corporal Jonathan; I had to admit his wife into the African hospital in Lusaka with pneumonia before our departure. It is the only testimonial that I can recall seeing and I still have the original.

I was due to return to the UK via Mombasa but my Commanding Officer managed to get dispensation for me to return home via Cape Town on RMS *Stirling Castle*. Jenny and I had been in frequent contact and by the time I got to Cape Town, although we had known each other for quite a short time, it was clear that we had reached 'an understanding'.

Just as I was about to depart I learned that my period of service was to be extended for six months because of the Korean War, and I ended up as a supernumerary medical officer in an Ordnance depot near Nottingham.

CHAPTER 5

Rural General Practice, 1950-2

AFTER ABOUT SIX WEEKS wasting time in Nottingham I got an SOS from my father. A young uncle running a single-handed general practice in the Machars of Galloway in south-west Scotland had taken his wife and daughters to the pantomime in Glasgow and had had a major heart attack. This would be in December 1950. The SOS was to ask if I could possibly get two or three days leave to temporarily hold the fort in this remote area. I was able to get away and arrived the following evening in my uniform. A very elderly retired general practitioner from some distance away had looked after the practice for the two days, he had done the evening surgery and on my arrival, he gave me the list of visits for the following day, put on his coat and left me.

The practice was based in Whithorn in the Burrowhead peninsula between Kirkcudbrightshire and the Mull of Galloway. In addition to the historic village of Whithorn it embraced the villages of Kirkinner, Garlieston, Sorbie, the Isle of Whithorn and the whole population in the country-side. The main occupations were farming, the creameries and fishing. There were some 2,500 patients in the practice and the nearest other doctors were some miles away in Wigtown and Port William. The Isle of Whithorn at the tip of the peninsula was not only a delightful fishing port but it was also traditionally associated with St Ninian, the first Christian missionary in Scotland, who settled in the area in

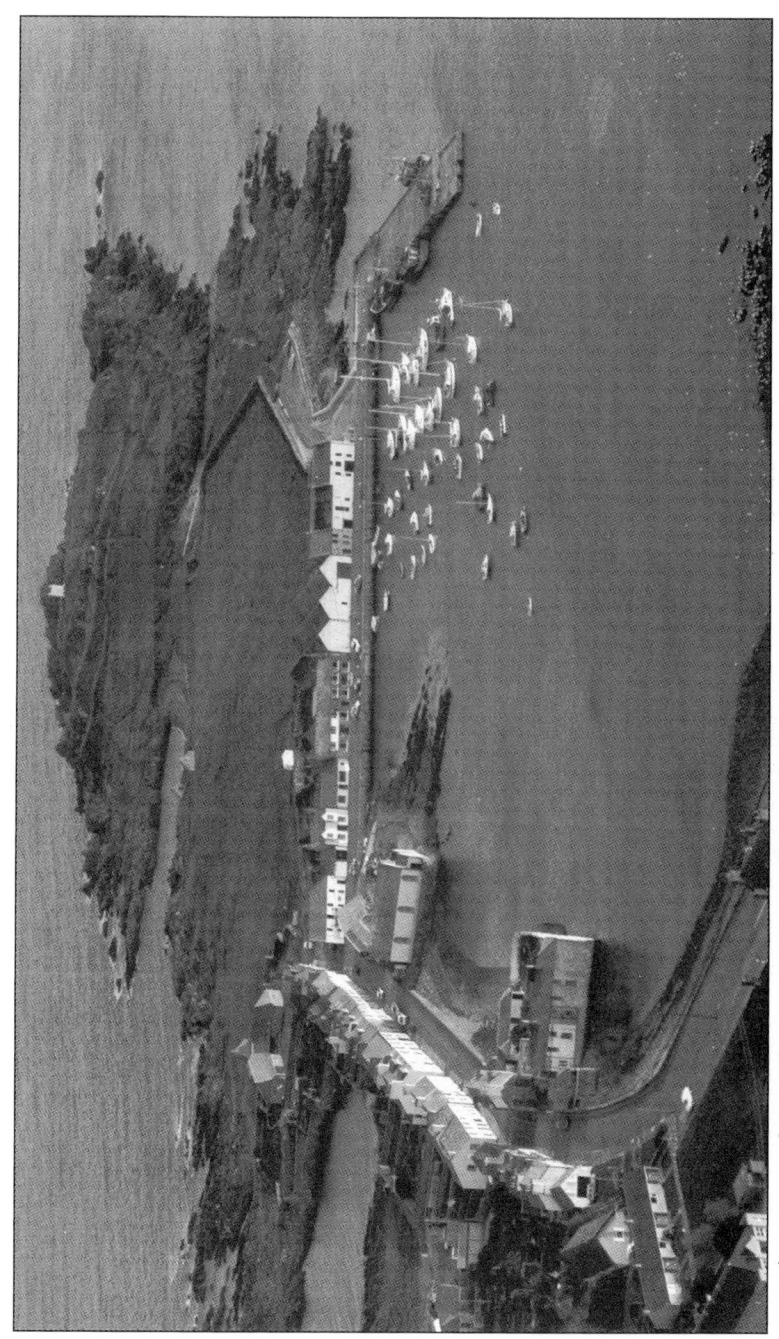

Aerial picture of the Isle of Whithorn where St Ninian settled around AD *400 and began to evangelise the southern Picts.*

the late fourth century on his return from Rome and set about evangelising the southern Picts. This was some 150 years before St Columba arrived in Iona from Ireland.

The uncle's family were to remain in Glasgow for a few days and I was quite alone but still full of youthful confidence and was not giving much thought to my rather awesome responsibility. There was a small cottage hospital in Stranraer but the main acute hospital was about 70 miles away in Dumfries.

During the first night I was called to two confinements. The family had gone to Glasgow by train and so uncle's car was in the garage; I had to get the young maid out of bed to find the car key, accompany me and show me the way. However Sister Robertson, a splendid district nurse from the Highlands, had preceded me in both homes and was in attendance when I got there.

I could not get away from Whithorn to return to the Army and with the help of the local MP I was eventually demobilised over the telephone. In those days a heart attack usually meant some six weeks in hospital and a long spell of convalescence, and so I was in charge and single handed for three to four months before my uncle returned to part-time work.

I reflect on the enormous respect in which the family doctor was then held. Within a few weeks I had been in almost every home because shortly after arrival there was a flu epidemic and then a measles epidemic, the latter being the first for about twenty years. Some time ago I enjoyed an after-dinner speech given by Dr Yellowlees of Aberfeldy in the Royal College of Physicians at the 50th reunion dinner of his 1941 Edinburgh class. He was remarking on how the esteem of the medical profession was so sadly declining but he went on to say that this was not true of the country doctor. Apparently a country general practitioner had been called out to certify the death of an elderly patient who had been ailing for some time. He finished his evening meal and went out to examine his patient. He said to his patient's wife, 'Jessie, I am afraid that Willie has slipped away.' With that Willie opened one eye and said, 'Jessie I'm no' away yet.' Jessie then admonished him and said, 'Wheesht Willie, the doctor kens best' ('Be quiet Willie, the doctor knows best')! That was the sort of regard which prevailed for the country doctor in 1951.

Looking back, I must have been rather busy. However the doctor was not pestered with trivia and if he was called out of his bed at night, which was not common, it was for something that needed his help. It could be something serious and urgent or the relatives were anxious and required reassurance.

I did a surgery morning and evening, Monday to Saturday and the Saturday evening attendance might be quite large if some had travelled in from the surrounding villages to see a good film at the local cinema! Home visits were requested in the mornings usually by telephone and I also divided domiciliary practice into three sections: the Isle of Whithorn and environs on Monday and Thursday afternoons, Garlieston on Tuesdays and Fridays and Sorbie on Wednesdays and Saturdays, and in each of these places, requests for visits were also left in a particular shop or the local Post Office. The visits were always made possible on that day although sometimes a few had to be done after the evening surgery. I do not remember any difficulty about getting urgent hospital admissions into the infirmary in Dumfries, or in getting outpatient appointments. The latter was helped by the senior physician and the senior surgeon from Dumfries each doing a clinic in Newton Stewart, some 18 miles away, once per month.

No doubt there were problems but fortunately I escaped any serious catastrophe. One Saturday evening after my surgery had finished, I was a little tired and also a little cross when a patient rang the front-door bell while I was having supper. I did however think from what I found that my visitor might have perforated a peptic ulcer and although the ambulance had to come from Newton Stewart he was on the operating table in Dumfries before midnight.

Midwifery was a major commitment but thankfully I always had Sister Robertson who was my main mentor and support. Indeed there were one or two occasions when I had to start some 'open' chloroform and Sister Robertson would keep it going while I scrubbed my hands hurriedly to get on with the business. Again I was lucky that this aspect of work, while sometimes a little worrying, did not cause too many difficulties.

Some three times a week letters had been exchanged with Jenny in Northern Rhodesia. My aunt once remarked that I must be obsessed with her, and indeed I was. Then in spring 1951, there was a major event – Jenny had returned home and I was able to get away briefly to meet her in London. Shortly afterwards she came to Whithorn and it became known that a young lady from Africa was coming to visit the doctor. It was said that most of the local populace, maybe two-thirds, had never been out of the area. I heard a rumour that a lot of my patients expected that the young lady would be black.

I went up to Newton Stewart to meet her off the train and a more gorgeous sight would be hard to imagine, albeit a little incongruous for Whithorn. She had on a mustard cape and a 1920s style hat with feathers dangling down to her waist. Then halfway down on the drive to Whithorn in the car she got out a long cigarette holder and lit a cigarette – and she was not a smoker. She was of course soon to be enormously popular, and to remain so. After this first visit I drove her down to Doncaster to meet my parents. On this occasion and on other short absences a locum had to be appointed and the first was an old friend who had been in my Edinburgh medical class (as had his wife).

In the summer, as I was now doing compulsory service in the Territorial Army as Medical Officer to the 5th Dumfries and Galloway Battalion KOSB, I had to do the first of four summer camps and I took the opportunity of driving down to Jenny's home in Hertfordshire. I had to explain to her father that Jenny and I wished to 'tie the knot' and he seemed to spend several minutes telling me about all the chaps that she might have had! However all was well and we had a delightful wedding in September in a church in St Albans and then a reception at Jenny's parents' farm at Wheathampstead. It was embarrassing to have received so many nice gifts from the Whithorn patients.

I have not so far mentioned that there was a high rate of births outside marriage, perhaps one in three, but it seemed to be acceptable and part of the local culture of the time. I used to pay pastoral visits to some of the elderly patients if I was passing near their homes although they might not have any immediate medical problem. I called on one particular lady in her eighties almost every week; we will call her Mary. Mary had had eight children and she told me that she was not sure of the father of any of them. However they had all

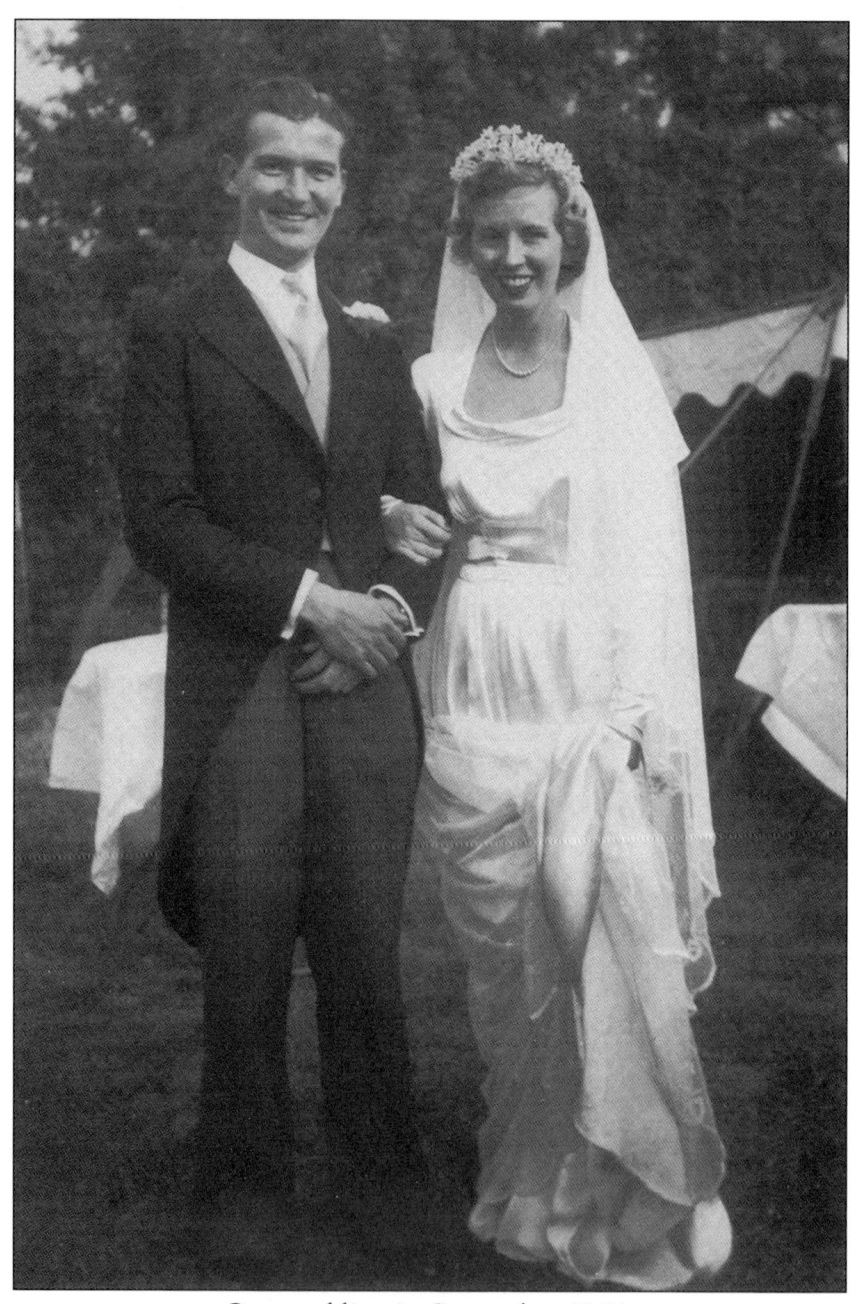

Our wedding in September 1951.

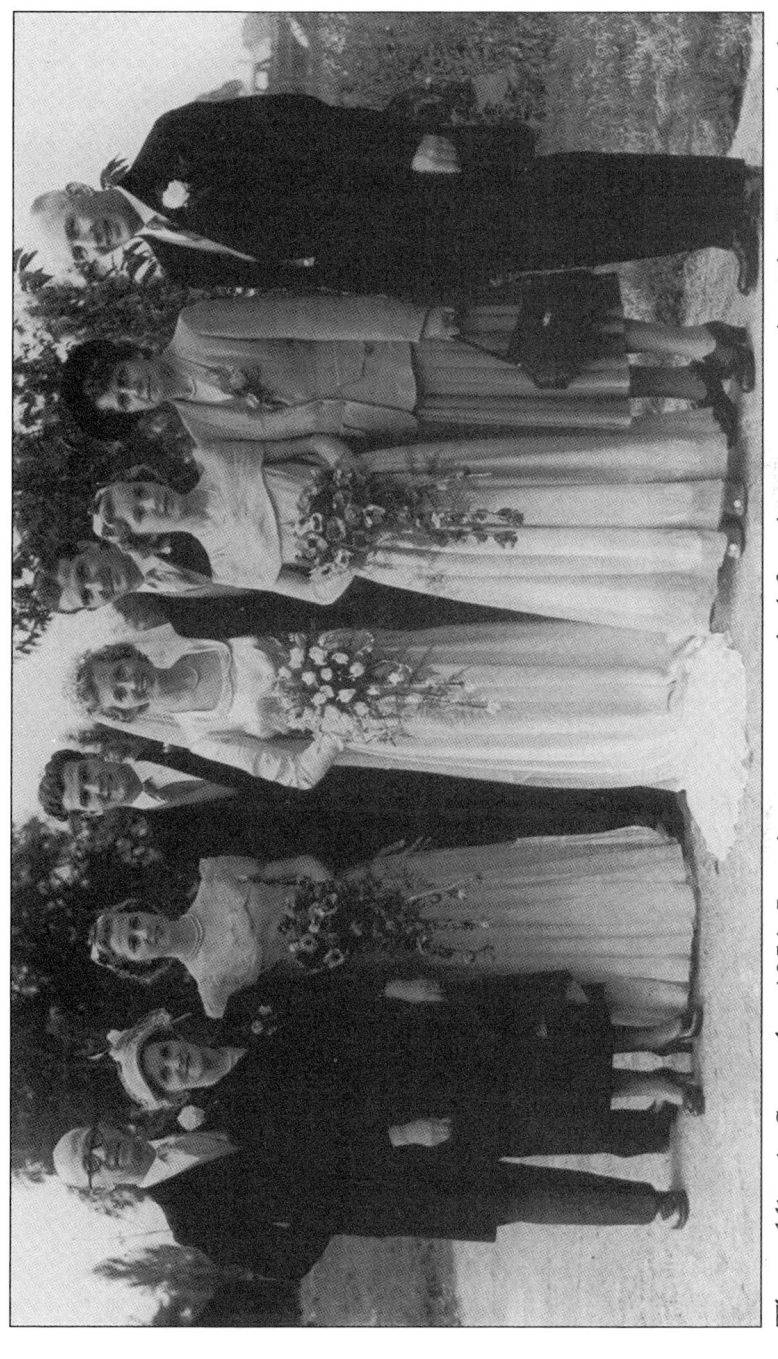

The wedding in September 1951. Jenny's parents are to the left and my parents to the right. Best man, brother James, is on Jenny's right and Nancy, Jenny's younger sister on his right. My sister, Elizabeth is in front of me.

done well and she lived with one son, and his family, who was a farm manager.

One afternoon I took my future wife with me on my round of home visits and we called on Mary who was delighted to entertain us with a cup of tea in the kitchen. Then she began to relate how she had brought up her children and had got to number three and could not afford the price of a pair of shoes to get the child to school. She was called in front of the school board and went in fear and trembling because she would be confronted at least by the Headmaster, the Laird, the Minister, the Town Clerk and the Bank Manager, and she fully expected that the child would be taken from her. She recalled that the first question was, 'Mary, how is it that you have managed the first two so well and this last yin's [one's] giving you so much trouble?' Mary responded by saying, 'How do you ken [know] it's the last yin when I dinna ken myself?' The Minister said, 'You have answered well, Mary,' and they all put their hands in their pockets to provide funds for the shoes.

I speak about Mary because I called to see her shortly before leaving to get married to thank her for the gift of a lovely water jug which we still have. She was in bed but jumped out, rolled back the mattress and gave me £2 in small silver coins which she had saved and which I was not allowed to refuse.

The first spell of marriage was of course delightful. My uncle was now back in harness and Jenny and I both began to feel that perhaps we would not wish to stay in Whithorn for the rest of our lives. It was then that I realised astonishingly that I seemed to have given no thought at all to my long-term career. This had been prompted a little earlier at my first Territorial Camp in the previous summer with the

Lowland Brigade when I discovered that several of my Edinburgh contemporaries had taken the Membership Examination of the Royal College of Physicians of Edinburgh. At that time, I did not seem to have any idea what the MRCP Ed was all about.

Rather to my uncle's displeasure we decided to move on and I thought that I should go and consult my former Professor of Medicine, Stanley Davidson. I had learned that he had two Assistant Lectureships in the University Department of Medicine which seemed to be the ideal appointment for someone at my stage, but I discovered that the posts were occupied and likely to be for some time. However the Professor indicated that I could not possibly know enough medicine to be considered for these posts and it would be a good plan to go for a year to the 'salt mines' in England. And so it was that I became a Senior House Officer in Kettering in Northamptonshire.

CHAPTER 6

The Later 1950s and the
Path of Postgraduate Development

KETTERING WAS A valuable next step. The General
Hospital was very well staffed. My duties with a newly
qualified House Officer, were to care for the patients in the
general medical ward, the children's ward and a nearby
convalescent hospital, take a full role in the medical
outpatient clinics and share in the work of the casualty
department. The consultant staff were mostly relatively
young graduates of London hospitals and there was excellent
rapport with the local general practitioners. In fact,
medically and indeed socially, we were all part of the one
community. I learned a great deal in Kettering, not least
from my consultant physician, the late Dr Partington.

I was due to spend one year in the Senior House Officer
post and after some nine months I felt it appropriate to
consult Professor Davidson again. Unfortunately the two
Assistant Lectureships were still occupied and the way ahead
was unclear. The sadness was compounded by the early
death of my father at the end of 1952. My mother was left
without comfortable financial resources; my brother was
now in medical school and my sister still in secondary
school.

Then, out of the blue, a letter came from Dr A. Rae
Gilchrist, a distinguished cardiologist in Edinburgh Royal
Infirmary. He had learned that I was trying to get back to

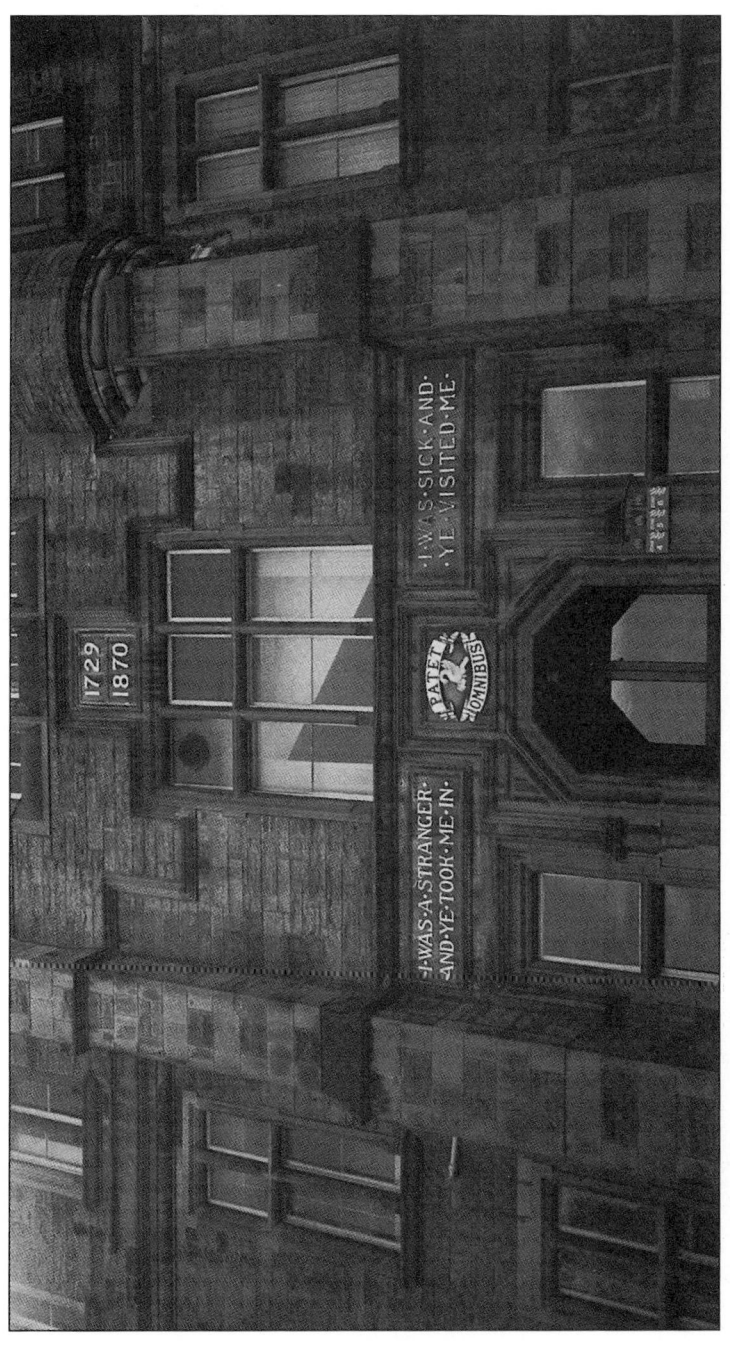

The Royal Infirmary of Edinburgh first opened with six beds in 1729 then moving to embrace 228 beds in 1741. The present one about to be replaced, opened in 1879. Famous quotation from St Matthew's gospel inscribed over main door.

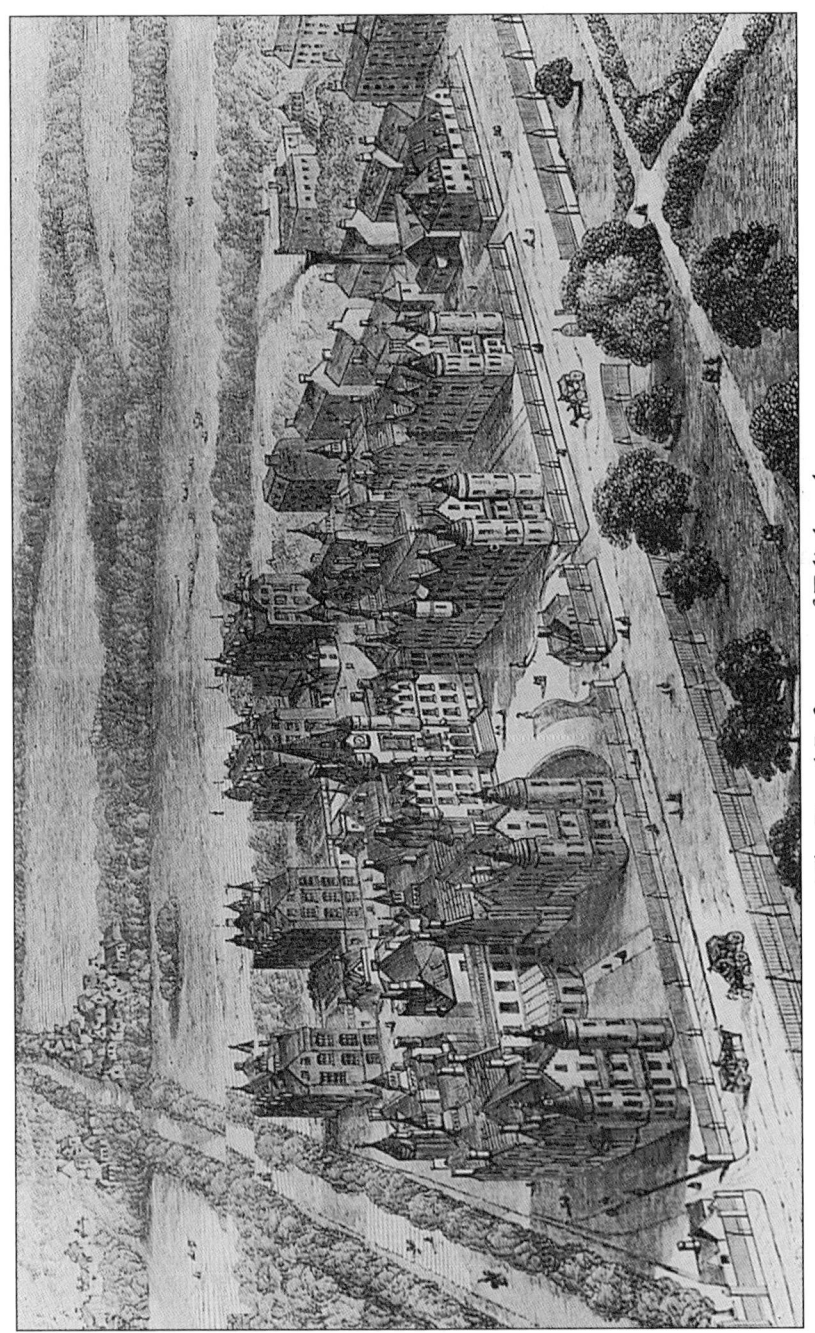

The Royal Infirmary of Edinburgh.

Edinburgh and a woman due to take one of his House
Officer posts in the Infirmary had let him down. I may say
that the woman was standing down to get married and she
and her husband were to become good family friends in
later years. I had to travel up to Edinburgh to see Dr
Gilchrist on the night train, my appointment was confirmed,
but I had to do it for twelve months! Fiscal matters were
quite troublesome. My stipend in Whithorn had been
£800 p.a., in Kettering £670 p.a. and now it was to be down
to £450 p.a. And our first son was to be born in March 1953,
my last month in Kettering.

However, back to Edinburgh it had to be. Jenny was
discharged from hospital on the day before we were due to
leave Kettering and I drove her down with new baby to her
parents' home in Hertfordshire in my Austin A40 Devon,
which I had been allowed to purchase as the doctor in
Whithorn when cars were in short supply. From memory it
had cost £506, a fortune at the time.

Jenny was to stay with her parents for some six weeks
while I went up to Edinburgh to start my House Officer job
and find a place to stay. I met her off the night train with
luggage and carrycot, and we repaired to our place of abode,
a fourth-floor tenement flat much like the one in which I
had spent my student days. I remember still her standing at
the bottom of the stairs as I proceeded upwards with some
of the baggage, and enquiring what she was doing, she
responded that she was waiting for the (non-existent) lift!
This particular housing complex in south Edinburgh was
built in the late 1800s.

Indeed four-storey blocks of tenement flats were very
much a feature of the old parts of Edinburgh and Glasgow.
In my own time as a student and on this return, I remember

well, that the coalman might have to carry upstairs ten or twenty bags of coal to be dumped in the coal bunker in the kitchen, inevitably with much dust. I heard a good story once about a lady spotting the coalman in the street below and shouting from a second-floor window, 'Coalman, two bags,' but he could not hear. Then after further attempts, she shouted in a very loud voice, 'Coalman, two bags, s'il vous plait.' This time he did hear and as he turned round he shouted, 'Mrs Mackenzie, you're not to get carried away with this European Community stuff, but seein' as ye ask, is it "cul de sac" or "à la carte"?'

This was a difficult year for us, my wife with new baby in a strange city and me in a busy House Officer post, living out for the first six months and compulsorily living in the Infirmary Doctors' Residence for the second six months. I was however in a very good team of caring doctors and teachers. At the end of my year in spring 1954, I was at last appointed to one of the two coveted Assistant Lecturer posts with Professor Davidson, and so my lifelong interest in haematology started now because this was Professor Davidson's favoured specialty. Then in January 1955 I became a research fellow for one year in the Rheumatic Diseases Unit at the Northern General Hospital, Edinburgh.

Also in January 1955, I passed the examination for the MRCP Ed. Two good friends, Bruce Paton and the late George Campbell also passed and on hearing the results, we celebrated over a half pint of beer in a pub in Rose Street behind the College of Physicians, then repaired to my home in Marchmont (still the tenement flat) for a banquet. I seem to remember that we each had a boiled egg!

The year at the Northern General Hospital was to be a

critical turning point. The unit was staffed by another outstanding team headed by the late Dr Ian Duthie from Aberdeen. I was introduced to strict research methods and to statistical analysis and a group of us managed to do some pioneer studies (later published) into the nature of the anaemia associated with rheumatoid arthritis. Then at the end of the year, I could hardly believe my good fortune – I was appointed to a full Lectureship with Professor Davidson.

It was now 1956. My clinical work was at Registrar level in the Professorial Medical Unit. The Medical Unit was essentially general medical wards, but with associated 'Blood Clinics' there was some emphasis on patients with blood disorders. Radioactive isotopes were now entering research techniques and I learned first how to label red blood cells with radioactive chromium (Chromium-51), for in-vivo investigation. This led to a particular interest in the haemolytic diseases, in which the red blood cells, which normally have a survival time of about three months, are destroyed abnormally rapidly. A related interest had to be the role of the spleen which in human beings after childhood is a fairly vestigial organ in the abdomen, but which usually has a role in the haemolytic anaemias. It can also be involved in quite a wide range of medical problems.

The interest in radioactive isotopes prospered with an excellent course on the subject in early 1957 in the Department of Medical Physics in Glasgow and then in early 1958 an outstanding course at the Atomic Energy Research Establishment in Harwell followed by three weeks of visits to research units in London hospitals.

In the autumn of 1957 I took the examination for Membership of the Royal College of Physicians of London.

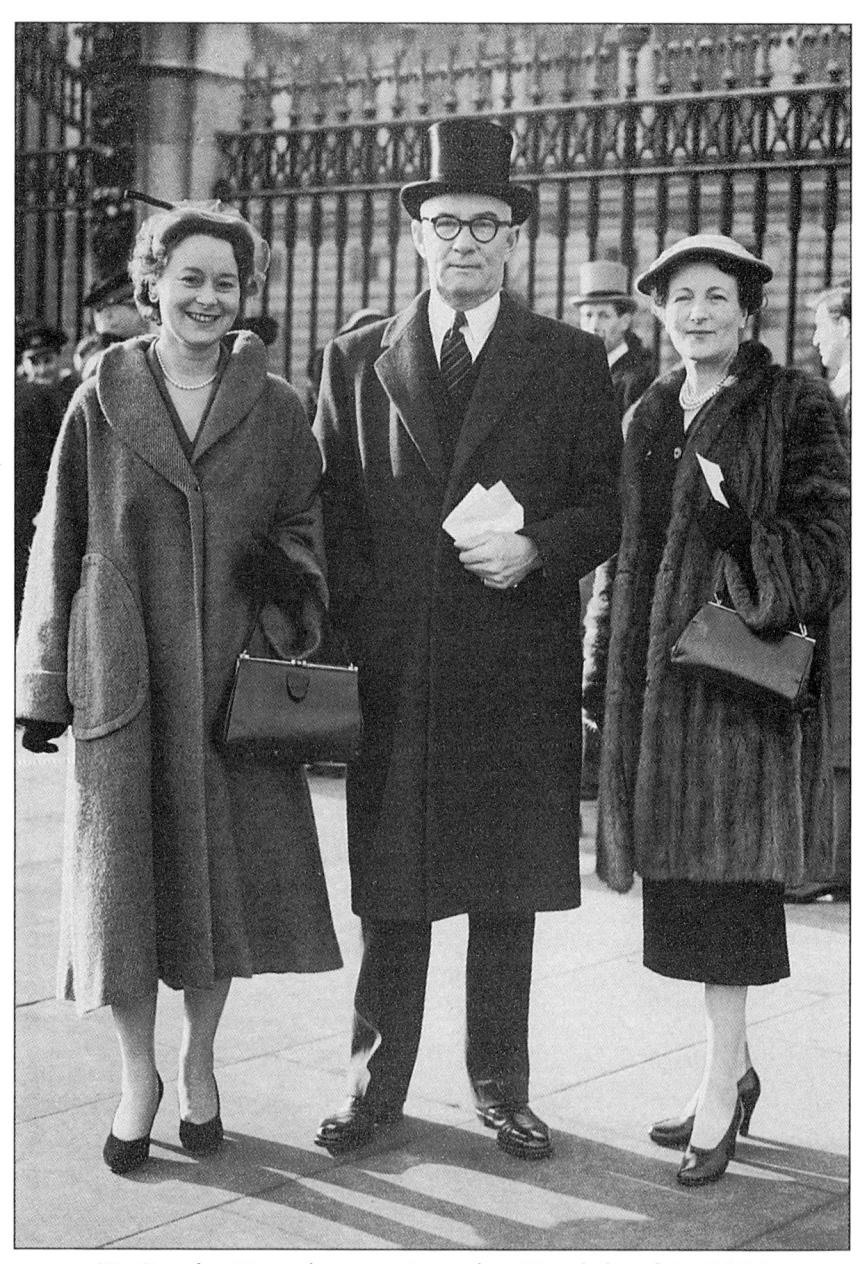

Sir Stanley Davidson receiving his Knighthood in 1956.
Lady Davidson is on his left.

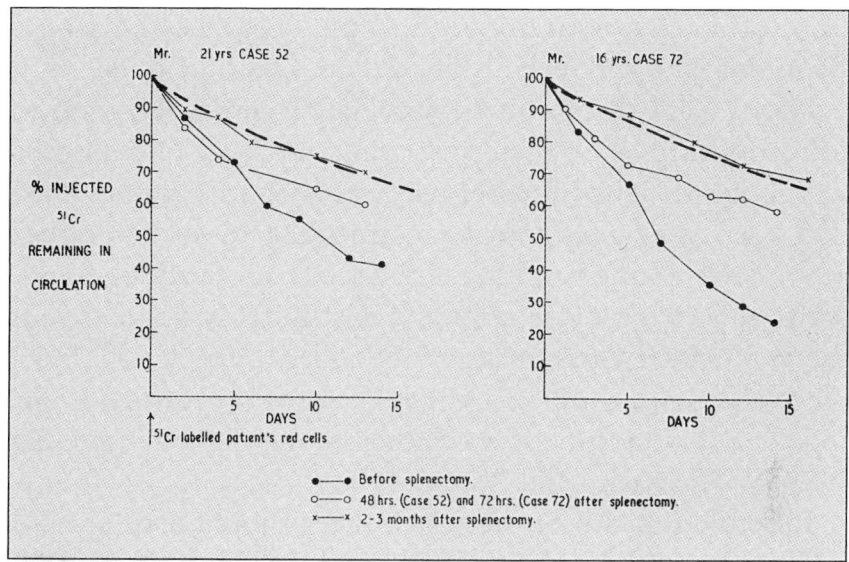

*Early studies using radioactive Chromium-51 (⁵¹Cr). The illustra-
tion shows the results in two patients with congenital spherocytosis
(an hereditary disease where the red blood cells have a shortened
survival time). Removal of the spleen produces gratifying results.
The interrupted line shows the normal survival time of labelled cells.
These are two of my best studies!*

Maybe this was not necessary, but there was a climate of
opinion at the time that one was unlikely to stand much
chance of a job south of the Wash without this qualification.
The London exam then was in three parts, spread over a
month. The pass rate was terrible. Of the 256 who started
with me, 22 got to the final oral examination in the College,
then in Trafalgar Square, and 21 passed.

When the 21 of us gathered at a later ceremony to receive
our diplomas, I was flattered when Professor McMichael
(see below) came over towards me. I presumed he was going
to offer congratulations and indeed he was, but he spoke

first to the chap standing next to me. That was Dr Roger Bannister who had recently broken the 4-minute mile!

When I got the result I immediately sent a telegram to Johannesburg. Jenny had just gone out for a few months with our two sons (number two was born in 1956) and had had a harrowing air journey controlling these two rather active boys. Jenny's mother and father had retired to South Africa to join her older sister and husband. I was able to join the family over Christmas and we added a happy stay down the Natal coast, south of Durban, before we returned home together. At that time it was rather a long flight stopping at Nairobi, Khartoum and Rome.

Recently it had been suggested that I should have a year's relevant training in the United States; many contemporaries were spending a year in the States in the 1950s. It was of course a very good medical and cultural experience, but some used to joke that it was to add BTA (Been To America) as a further qualification after their names. The famous Memorial Sloan Kettering Cancer Center in New York seemed ideal for me and I was fortunate to get a placement as a research fellow and also a Fulbright Scholarship. The year there was to begin in autumn 1958.

Professor Davidson, now Sir Stanley, was due to retire in 1959 but in summer 1958 he had a special dinner for the full-time lecturers who had been appointed to his department during his professional career. He had started as the first full-time Professor of Medicine in Scotland in Aberdeen in 1930; then he moved to Edinburgh in 1938. Although Sir Stanley had had large numbers of doctors attached to his two departments, particularly after the Second World War, many of whom had reached high places, surprisingly he had had only seven full-time lecturers and

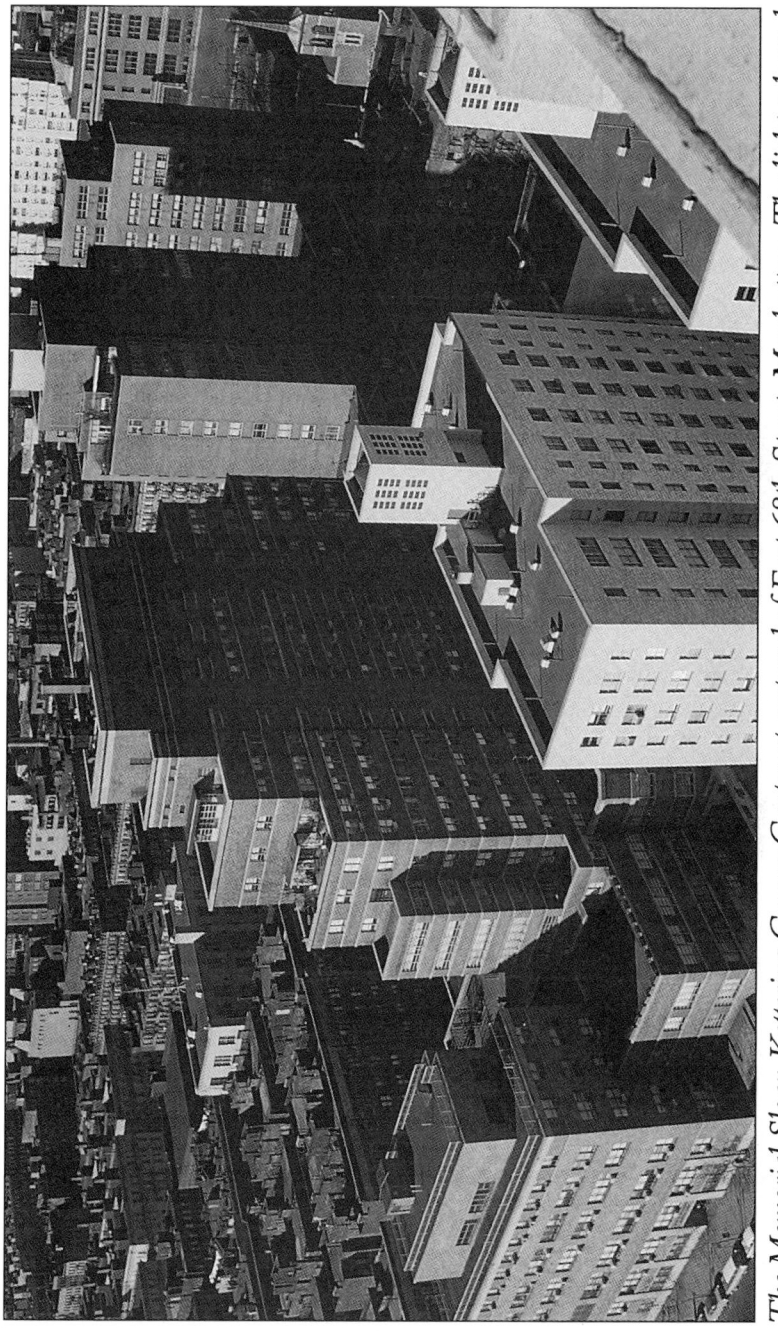

The Memorial Sloan Kettering Cancer Center at east end of East 68th Street, Manhattan. The light coloured building in the foreground was our apartment building.

they were all able to attend the retirement dinner. It was a memorable occasion indeed.

Those present were John McMichael, Professor of Medicine at the Royal Postgraduate Medical School in London, I.G. Hill, Professor of Medicine in Dundee, H.W. Fullerton, Professor of Medicine in Aberdeen, L.J. Davis, Professor of Medicine in Glasgow, J.G. McCrie, the first full-time medical Dean in the country and based in Sheffield, R.H. Girdwood, later to be Professor of Therapeutics in Edinburgh, and me.

I could not understand why Professor, later Sir Derrick Dunlop, a close colleague of Sir Stanley, but never on his staff, was included. Derrick was there to entertain our wives and this he did at a separate circular table at the window. Sir John McMichael's speech of reminiscences rang a few bells in all of us.

The trip to New York was on the *Mauretania* and the two boys enjoyed it as much as Jenny and I did. We met lots of interesting people and we particularly enjoyed the company of a schoolmaster from New England and his delightful wife.

The Memorial Sloan Kettering Cancer Center comprised a private hospital, a central large research institute and a state hospital occupying a full city block between East 67th and East 68th Street. York Avenue bordered the east side of the block and across the avenue were the Rockefeller Institute and New York Hospital. Our apartment block was over the road in East 68th Street and we were of course in the heart of Manhattan.

We had planned that our number one son would go to the United Nations School particularly as the primary classes were close by. However on the eve of the first day of term I

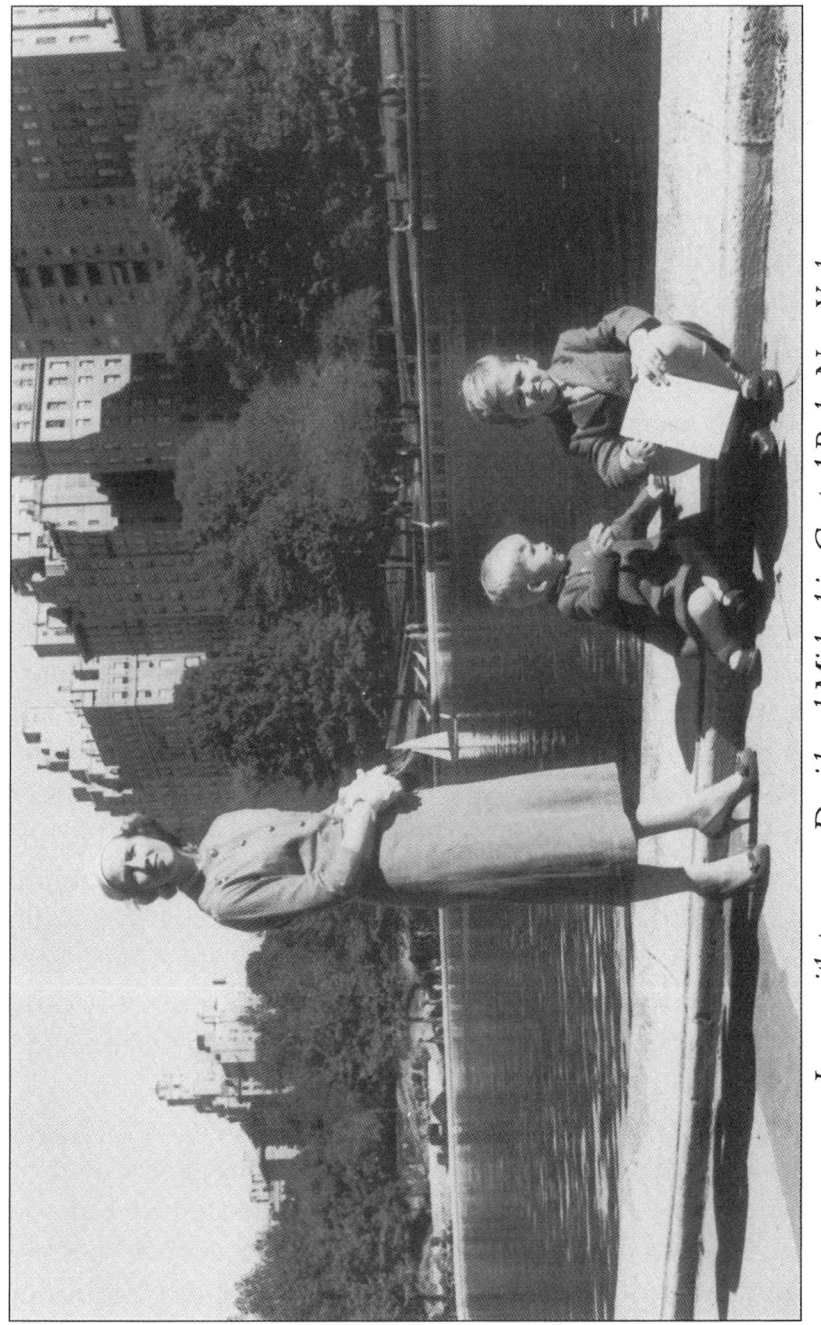

Jenny with two sons David and Michael in Central Park, New York.

discovered that the term's fee was almost as much as my whole year's income! He ended up having a very good year at PS 183 in East 67th Street. Indeed his teacher was to come and visit us in Edinburgh a few years later.

The clinical and research experience in the midst of outstanding staff, many of world renown, was to have lifetime interest. I was able to see a wide variety of malignant diseases, particularly leukaemias and lymphomas. Many chemotherapeutic agents dating from the trials with nitrogen mustard in the Second World War, were now on the horizon but they were not yet being used so effectively as they are today. My research was committed to looking into the red cell survival time in malignant lymphoma and also adding to the Institute's extensive study of organ involvement in the lymphomas; I was assigned to a detailed analysis of their pathological records of kidney involvement.

I have mentioned my early upbringing in the Plymouth Brethren and this continued through my student days. Jenny was confirmed in the Church of England and we came together in the Church of Scotland, which was how we came to be regular attendees at Madison Avenue Presbyterian Church. Here there was of course an enormous congregation, often with two 'houses' on a special Sunday morning. A most interesting finding was that the highly regarded preaching minister, Dr David Read, had had his earlier days in Greenbank Church in Morningside, Edinburgh.

On one evening each week Dr Read and his wife held a gathering for young people in his penthouse apartment on Fifth Avenue. Apart from supper and gossip, we enjoyed some Scottish country dancing. It was here that we met two young men, one married, and they were both beginning

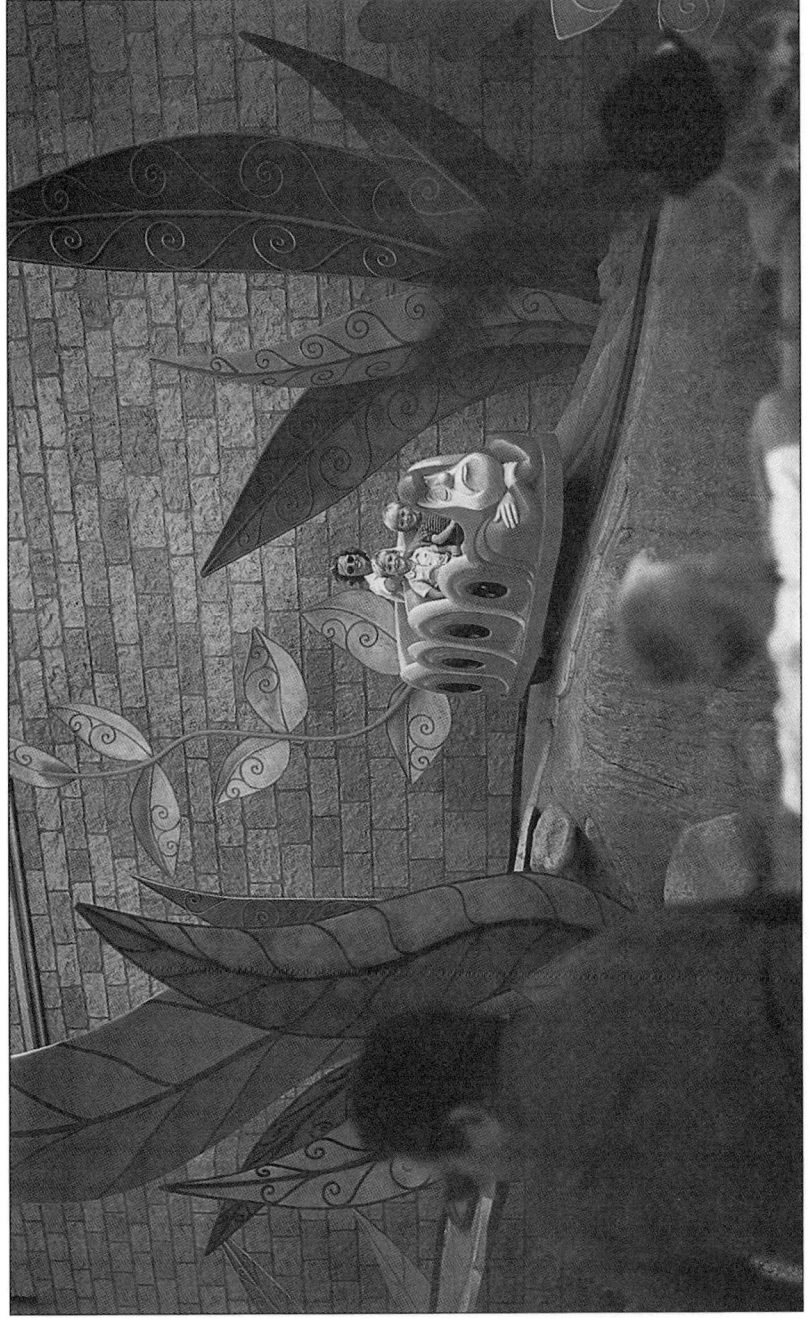

Jenny with the two boys in Disneyland.

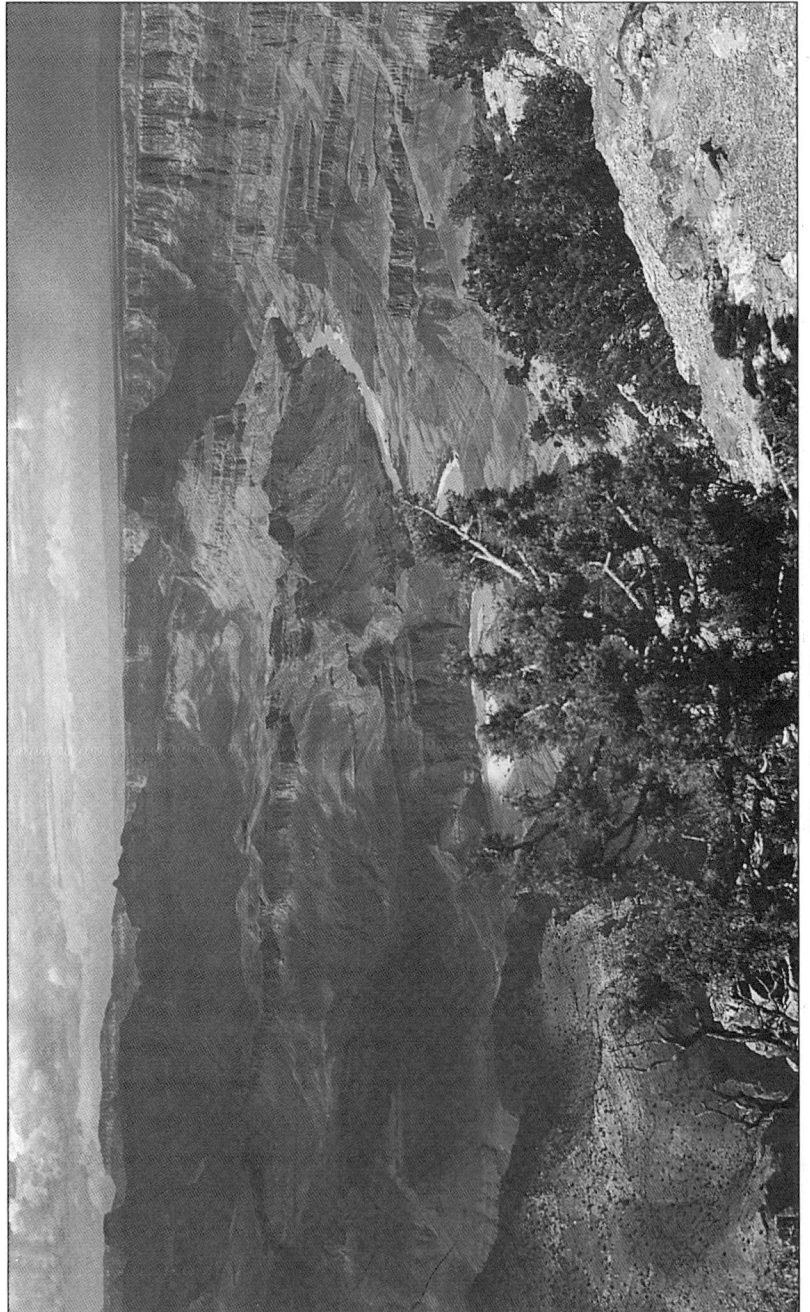

The Grand Canyon, USA.

their careers in the Wall Street Bank, J.P. Morgan and Co. I will refer to them as Mr R and Mr B.

Mr R, who visited us with his wife in Edinburgh recently, is now a retired Vice Chairman of J.P. Morgan and Co. He thought that as we did not have a car in New York, we should borrow his for a tour during our last month before returning to Edinburgh; it was a VW Beetle. I am somewhat embarrassed to recount that with our two little boys, we did 9,000 miles via Niagara Falls, Chicago, Rapid City, Denver (where my MRCP Ed contemporary Bruce Paton was now a cardiological surgeon), Salt Lake City, San Francisco, Disneyland, Baja California, Tijuana, Mexicali, Grand Canyon, Oklahoma, New Orleans, Augusta, Washington and back to New York. There were numerous incidents which we still recall. On one occasion in a small town in the far west a lady in the shop was flabbergasted when she saw that the Beetle had a New York number plate and called her husband to see it. When she learned that we were from Edinburgh I remember her husband exclaiming, 'Good old Edinburgh on the Clyde'. Perhaps the worst experience was after we had all had a swim in the Great Salt Lake in Utah. As we were returning to the car, shivering in the early evening, I could not recall what had happened to the car key. I had in fact put it in the pocket of my swimming trunks and it was now at the bottom of the lake! It took quite a long time to get a young locksmith out from Salt Lake City, a good few miles away, but in a few minutes all was well.

The two little boys behaved very well but were anxious that when we got to California we would stay in a motel 'with heated swimming pool and television in every room'. This we did, for two or three nights, in Santa Barbara. However on the point of departure, when I got into the car,

I could not see very well and realised that I was not wearing my spectacles. This meant searching our bedroom and all our luggage but without success. Eventually Jenny saw the spectacles looking at her from the deep end of the swimming pool. I had obviously dived in wearing them in the early morning!

Mr B wrote to me in Edinburgh in the middle of the 1960s when he was Monsieur le Directeur of J.P. Morgan and Co. in Paris, to ask if I could give him a medical overhaul. This I did – and what was my fee? I have never been in fee-paying practice, but in any case one would never dream of charging a friend or a colleague. I had to say courteously not to be ridiculous. A few days later we received a crate of Chateau Lynch Bages, which in our naivety we drank like Coca Cola, and also a Methuselah (equivalent to eight bottles) of champagne. Jenny thought that we should keep the champagne for number one son's 21st birthday some years ahead. We did in fact 'blow it' three nights later and had a grand party.

One other episode remains clear in my memory. During our year in Manhattan, the New England schoolmaster and his wife whom we had met on the *Mauretania* took us out one night to dinner at a most luxurious restaurant and it was a great pleasure to renew their friendship. However, I was troubled by my thinking that we might have difficulty in ever returning their kindness. Then I remembered his saying that he was going to be attending a summer school at Columbia University in New York. With much research I secretly discovered that he would be staying with his wife's family in Manhattan and it was arranged that I would entertain him one evening. At this time my wife and the boys had escaped the New York summer humidity to stay with friends in Cape Cod. I decided to take my friend to the famous Rainbow Room at the top of the Rockefeller Center. I had never been there and felt that perhaps neither had he.

I telephoned the head waiter to reserve a table and heard the most Scottish voice imaginable. I asked where in Scotland he had come from and he told me it was a town, Saltcoats on the west coast. I told him that I had come from Scotland, and he hastened to say, 'Well the first thing is, it is far too expensive for you here. Come here first and give your friend a couple of cocktails; then go down to street level to a nice wee restaurant where I used to be the head waiter. You'll get a grand dinner there for half the price.'

I did as instructed and on arrival at the Rainbow Room with my friend, I was greeted by name as if I was a regular customer. We were given a table at the window with a marvellous view and received a couple of cocktails 'on the house'. Then we went down to the street level where we did have a 'grand dinner' and also with a bottle of wine 'on the house'.

Years later, quite by chance, Jenny and I met the schoolmaster and his wife in Harrods!

I seem to be recalling many fiscal matters but these were in fact rather impecunious days. Through the good offices of my Wall Street companions I had actually put my wife's return boat fare on the New York Stock Exchange with a happy outcome. We sailed home on the *Queen Mary* in September 1959. The children for some time retained memories of our visit. On passing through Waterloo Station on our way back to Edinburgh number two son was desperate to enjoy a hamburger and a coke!

CHAPTER 7

Commitment to Clinical Medicine, Teaching and Research in the University Sphere

RETURN TO EDINBURGH was not easy. I had been attracted to one or two possible appointments in the United States but in those days on an Exchange Visitor's visa one had to return to base for two years. I think also that I was concerned not to desert my widowed mother. A major factor was however that my mentor, Sir Stanley Davidson, had retired and the new Professor was interested in cardio-respiratory research which was not a branch of medicine in which I felt well informed. However, Professor Donald, despite his relatively small number of established staff allowed me to continue with my interest in haematology and oncology.

In the 1950s, training posts, and indeed consultant posts, were in relatively short supply and so most of us spent a long time in a variety of appointments but this led to a good general grounding and wide experience. Indeed the career prospects were so uncertain that large numbers of skilled doctors emigrated to North America, Australia and other parts of the Commonwealth, a choice made by approximately one third of my own class. Eventually in 1963, fifteen years after graduating, I was appointed Senior Lecturer in the University Department of Medicine and Honorary Consultant Physician in the Royal Infirmary of Edinburgh.

But just before this, I met Sir Stanley Davidson in the town. He had started a textbook of medicine in 1952 which had already become a world best seller and multiple editions later, it still is. In 1959 the first visible chromosome abnormalities in man had been described. The very first, a sex chromosome abnormality causing a condition known as Klinefelters syndrome, had been reported from Edinburgh by Drs Jacobs and Strong. The one related to Down's syndrome (mongolism) followed shortly afterwards. Sir Stanley said, 'Richmond, we are needing to have a chapter on genetics in the book and as you won't know anything about genetics, you had better write it!' This I took on, somewhat reluctantly, for the next three editions, but by this time advances were accelerating so rapidly that I was getting out of my depth.

Later I shared the chapter on liver disease for several editions, indeed until retirement. On one occasion I had an amusing exchange with a very senior officer in the Royal Army Medical Corps (RAMC), and he was telling me what a splendid primer Davidson's book was and how it was widely used in the RAMC. He went on to say, however, that there was one section in it that was absolutely awful. 'In fact,' he said, 'it is absolutely bloody awful.' It was a paragraph or two on a condition known as 'leptospirosis'. I had to respond by saying that that was most unfortunate because I happened to write it! It is an important if relatively rare infection in the UK but a more common cause of infections, many of them minor, in south-east Asia. My army officer critic had seen quite a lot of it and had become an expert on the subject.

Also in 1963 I was elevated to Fellowship of the Royal College of Physicians of Edinburgh and fairly soon afterwards became a regular examiner in the MRCP (Ed).

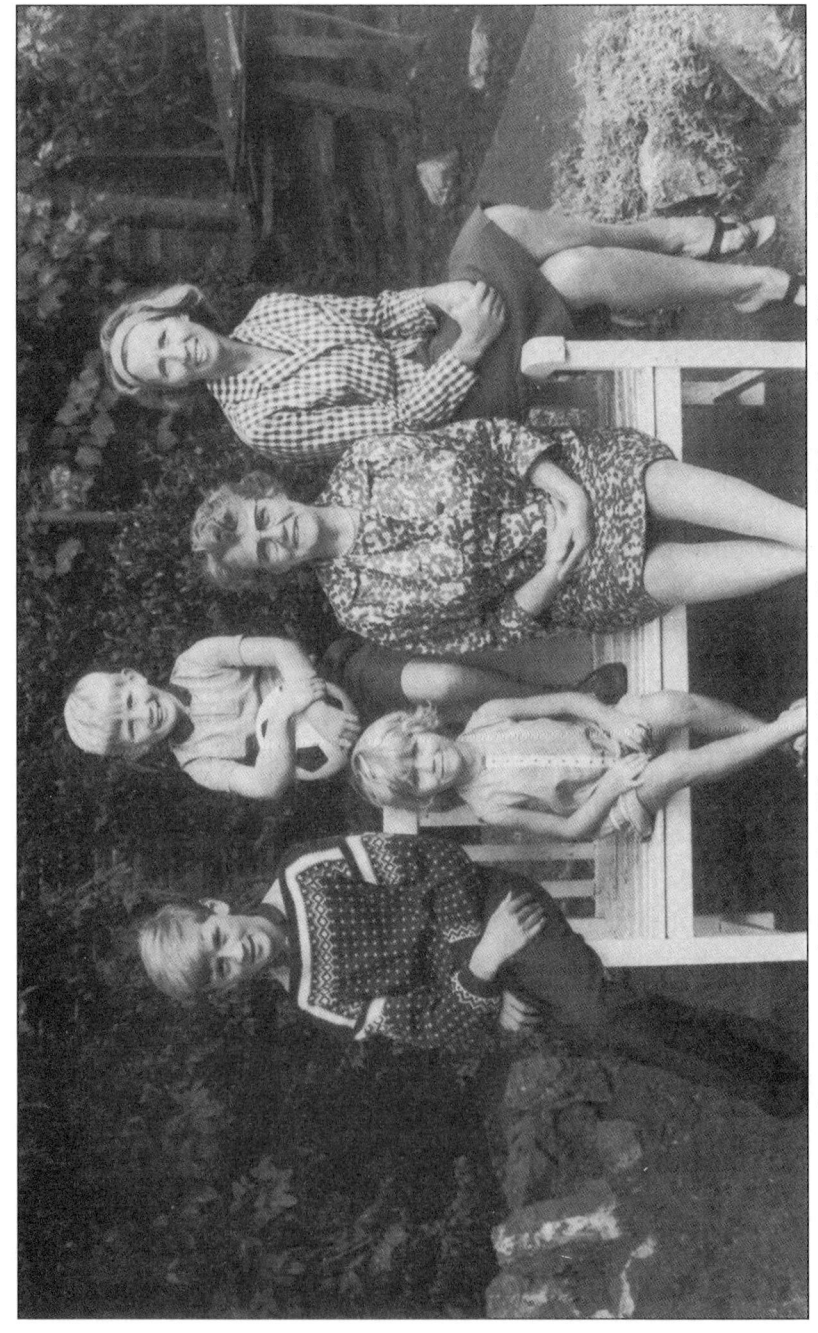

Family picture with David, Michael, Virginia, Granny Richmond and Jenny, 1964.

University medicine has gradually become more and more immersed in valuable research. However, in Edinburgh at that time, the Professorial Medical Unit had two wards in the Infirmary comprising sixty acute general medical beds and it took its turn along with the other five medical units to be twenty-four hours 'on take' for emergency admissions, Sundays being done in rotation. The average number of admissions was fifteen to twenty, less than at the present time. The problems covered the whole range of medicine and so most of us had to preserve ourselves as 'general physicians'. Neurology had for some forty years been a distinct specialty and Infectious Diseases for longer. Dermatology, ENT and Ophthalmology had also been distinct entities. Specialism was however now extending, particularly in Respiratory Medicine, Cardiology, Endocrinology, Gastroenterology and Renal Medicine.

I continued my interest in haematology and many general medical admissions had a haematological component. But, sadly for me haematology was increasingly becoming a laboratory-based discipline. My own research continued however in the haemolytic diseases, platelet disorders and the use of radioactive isotopes.

In 1965, I had a four-month visit to Makerere University in Kampala, Uganda. This had arisen because Professor Ian Hill (my physician chief in the Deaconess Hospital in 1948-9) had passed through, visiting the then Professor of Medicine, John Tulloch, who had been Senior Registrar with Dr Gilchrist in 1953, when I had been the House Physician. It is a small world! Professor Hill had been amazed by the number of Ugandan patients with enormous spleens. In the healthy adult, the spleen is about the size of the palm of the hand and weighs some 125gms. The enormous spleens in the Ugandans were having very adverse effects. Apparently it was suggested that Richmond would be most interested. There had already been some studies of 'big spleen disease' from places like Papua New Guinea, but so far there had been little investigation of the problem in a homogeneous group of patients.

It was a great privilege to be joined by Dr Roger Williams from London, a noted authority on liver disease which is often accompanied by splenic enlargement. We each had a supporter, Roger being accompanied by his technician and me by my research fellow in Edinburgh, Dr Keith Donaldson, now in British Columbia.

At that time Makerere University was an academic oasis. The Mulago Hospital, the teaching hospital, had been built just before Uganda gained independence. President Obote was then in charge of the country and everything seemed to

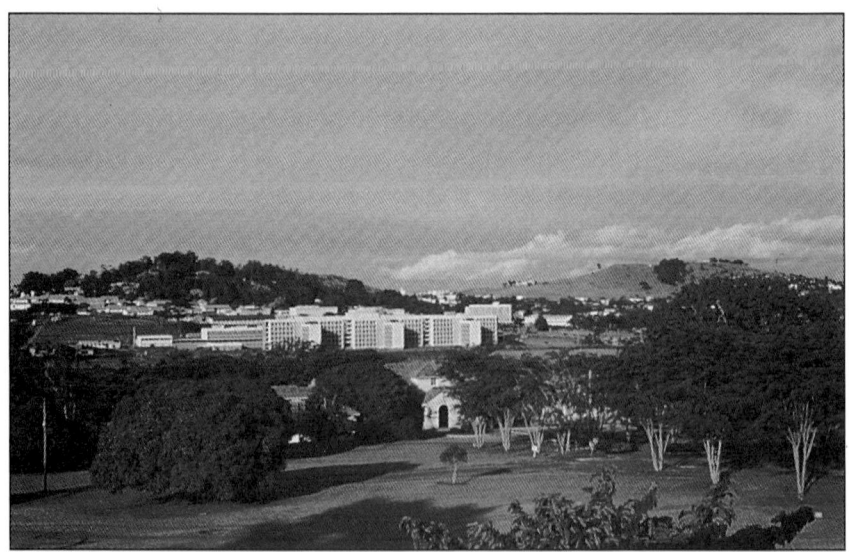

Mulago Hospital, Uganda with laboratory departments in the background.

be going well. There were excellent British academic staff and a visiting American Professor of Medicine. Ugandan undergraduate and postgraduate students of high calibre were emerging. When I returned in 1971 on a teaching visit, Idi Amin had just displaced President Obote and signs of the disintegration that was to follow were already apparent.

I do however have one strong memory of this later visit. There was a graduation ceremony for very many happy students, in a large marquee. At the end, the Vice-Chancellor installed Idi Amin as Chancellor of the University. Idi Amin's acceptance speech started with his reading from some prepared text and he was soon struggling with long English words. Shortly he screwed up his piece of paper, threw it over his shoulder and proceeded to speak 'off the cuff'. I remember his saying to the new graduates something along the lines, 'Now you lot are highly privileged and it is your job to get back into the bush and help your less privileged brothers.' Nothing could have been more appropriate for the occasion. Sadly, however, we were later to learn that the Vice-Chancellor had disappeared, then the Lord Chief Justice and so on.

Our research showed that the very large spleens in our patients were causing profound anaemia and thrombo-cytopenia (low platelet numbers) due to 'pooling' of blood in the spleen outwith the general circulation. The spleen was removed in a few patients with excellent return of a normal blood picture. In one patient the 'big spleen' actually weighed over 5kg. We would never have considered this procedure in later years when it was discovered that removing the spleen could have a significant effect on the immune system, not only in children, but could leave any patient vulnerable to particular bacterial infections.

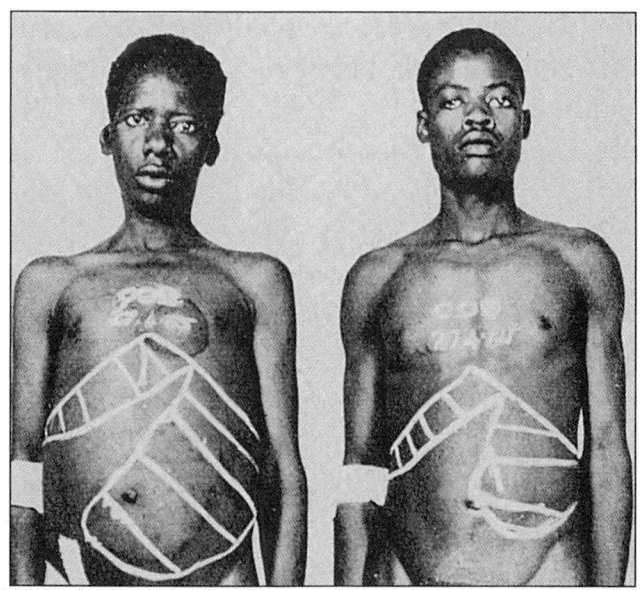

Two male patients with 'big spleen disease',
now known as tropical splenomegaly syndrome.

Moreover it was believed then and subsequently confirmed, that 'big spleen disease', later to be known as 'tropical splenomegaly syndrome', was due to chronic and recurrent malarial infection, particularly in persons who had immigrated from non-malarious areas. Also it was found that the 'big spleen' could be reduced in size by administering antimalarial therapy over many months.

The visit to Uganda was memorable also because of excursions to the north to game reserves, the origin of the White Nile and the Murchison Falls, and also to the southwest, the latter apparently rather a dangerous area for tourists nowadays.

One excellent colleague was Dr Francis Lothe, a Norwegian but a Sheffield graduate who was the Chief Government Pathologist. Although there were strange

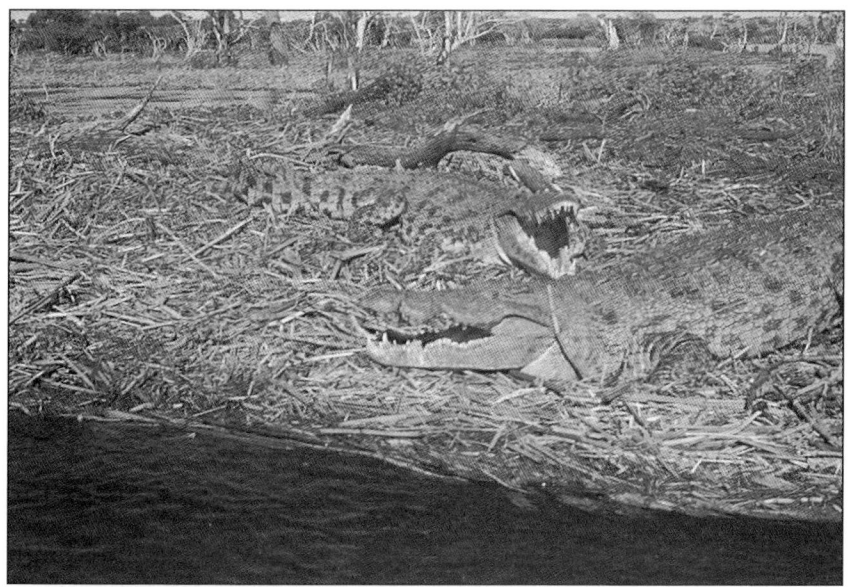

Crocodiles on the White Nile, uncomfortably close to our boat.

diseases in Uganda apart from tropical disorders, for example a lot of hepatitis B, there was absolutely no question of HIV infection or AIDS which is now devastating the country. In our last week Francis asked if I would look after the pathology service while he took his wife to Kenya to take part in the Ladies' Open Golf Championship, which she won. Mrs Lothe came from the Sheffield area and later their two daughters were to become students in the Sheffield Medical School.

I should not have deserted my wife for so long because we now had three children, having added a daughter in 1961. I did however have her permission to set off with a return ticket to South Africa which allowed me to stop off in Uganda.

I went first to the new medical school in Salisbury,

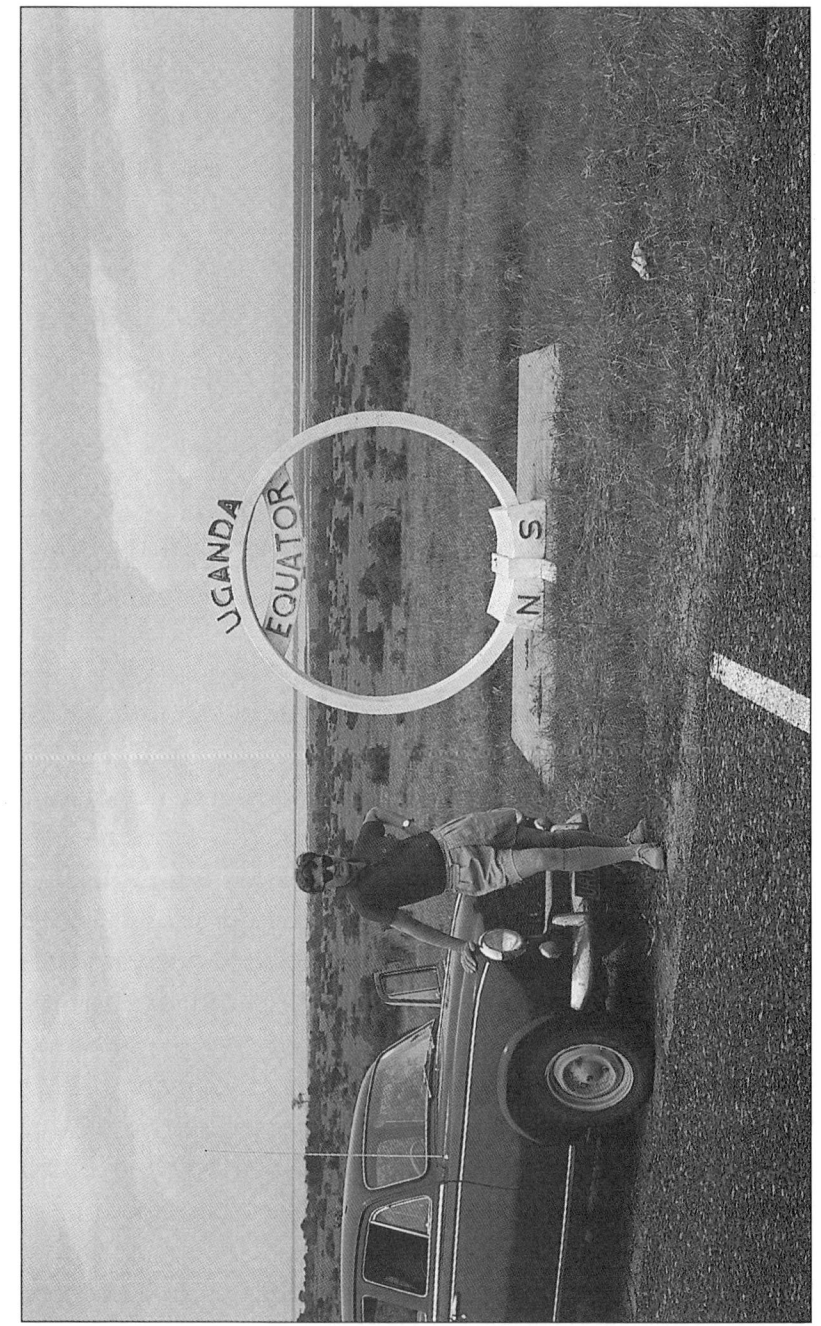

The author standing on the equator in south-west Uganda.

Southern Rhodesia where my opposite number and colleague in the Deaconess Hospital in 1948-9, Lindsay Davidson, was now Professor of Medicine. Then I went on to Johannesburg to visit Jenny's two sisters who had married and settled there, and on for a brief visit to Durban to see George Campbell who had taken the MRCP (Ed) with me in 1955.

George had me out of bed early next morning to join him on his round of patients in local nursing homes. While on our round he got a call to go and see a doctor in Empangeni in Zululand who was thought to have had a heart attack. We left in a little four-seater aeroplane from a strip at Umhlanga Rocks and nearly crashed taking off. We did a cardiograph (ECG) on the doctor and confirmed that he had had a heart attack; after doing what we could, we set off back to Durban.

George was a great authority on tropical fish and our next destination was the Oceanographic Institute in Durban where he had some research appointment. The place had large fish tanks, full of large fish and George's interest was to get the fish out of the tanks, sedate them in some way and do cardiographs on them. The fish heart has only three chambers compared with the four in humans and so the cardiographs looked bizarre. I came away with a cardiograph from a shark which unhappily I seem to have mislaid.

Next day I was back in Johannesburg and I wanted to see a girl student whom I had sent out from Edinburgh to do her 'elective' at Baragwanath hospital. She happened to have been assigned to the wards of the late Dr Leo Shamroth, one of the world authorities on electrocardiography and whose books are highly regarded. He kindly took me out for lunch and I was of course moved to tell him about the doctor in

Zululand and the visit to the fish tanks and then I showed him the shark's ECG. I do not think that he had been following my story because he thought the strange ECG was from the doctor and he exclaimed, 'My God, you did not dare to leave him did you?' or words to that effect!

Still feeling guilty about my long absence my air ticket included a brief stop in Rome on my return journey. In 1965 the VC10 landed in Nairobi and then Khartoum and having left Johannesburg one evening, I woke up early next morning over the 'toe' of Italy. By lunchtime I had already done most of Rome, a very beautiful city.

Back home to the bosom of the family, Jenny was in good heart and many friends had given her much support. I must have had some funds left over from my 'per diem' allowance and shortly we were having a grand holiday at the splendid Sandbanks Hotel at Poole in Dorset.

I did not ever leave my family for so long again. There was a brief visit in 1967 back to the Sloan Kettering Institute in New York for some award, going on to visit a colleague in Johns Hopkins Hospital, Baltimore. The Baltimore colleague was soon to be Professor of Medicine in the University of Florida in Gainesville. He came for a spell to Edinburgh and then in 1969 he asked me to hold the fort for him in Gainesville for a couple of weeks which was another rewarding experience. During this visit I was taken to Cape Canaveral where in the distance one could see a rocket in place; it was to be the one that took the first men to land on the moon. The return home took me via the Bahamas because I wished to call on a physician, John Lunn, who was doing well. He was an Edinburgh graduate and he had been a research fellow with me in the early 1960s; he was the first Bahamian to get the MRCP (Ed).

Between these digressions, I was still enjoying my clinical work and research in Edinburgh. I had to give quite a few lectures but on most mornings, my particular pleasure was challenging bedside teaching. Indeed I was beginning to realise that medical education of the undergraduate and young postgraduate was my main preoccupation. I think that this was emphasised because in the middle 1960s the Faculty of Medicine had commissioned a few of us at non-professorial level from different departments to review and revise the undergraduate curriculum. This we did to try and take account of recent trends and changing emphasis and our report was received with generally favourable comment. Also in the late 1960s I had been charged with preparing MCQ (multiple choice question) papers for the Final MB Examination in Medicine. These papers traditionally contained sixty questions each with five possible answers. This shortly led to sharing in confidence our MCQ examinations with two other medical schools over a five-year period. One interesting consequence was that we were able to get some idea of the weaknesses and strengths of each medical school's teaching.

Hospital administration in the late 1960s seemed to run smoothly. In the Edinburgh Royal Infirmary there was a physician/superintendent, a senior male hospital secretary and a matron each with supporting clerical staff. Many of us did a spell on the Board of Management but this was simply a multidisciplinary advisory group without executive function which met once per month. Administration and bureaucracy nowadays has exploded and is the subject of much complaint.

Around the same time, there were two government reports that were to have very important consequences. The

Salmon Committee's report of 1966 on senior nurse staffing structure had a lasting impact. I hope that I have already been able to emphasise the critical relationship between the doctor and the nurse. Many of us regret the demise of the traditional ward sister and of the matron, both of whom were now to be known by numbers. But most importantly the changes meant that the good caring ward sister had to contemplate becoming an administrator in order to gain promotion and some improvement in her modest stipend.

The report of the Royal Commission on Medical Education (the Todd Report) was presented to Parliament in April 1968 after three years' deliberation. Its many recommendations were far reaching and a few are worth highlighting. Accepting that practical instruction needed to be incorporated at an early stage of training the requirement for apprenticeship was seen to be now mainly at postgraduate level but it was still largely haphazard and disorganised. With the great growth of knowledge it was felt that all doctors, general practitioners as well as consultants, should continue to gain expertise. The undergraduate period should seek to produce not a finished doctor as in the 1940s, but a broadly educated person ready for further training and continuing education. As a result of recent and unforeseeable future advances, changes in the pattern of medical services and the rising demands of society the report also concluded that there would need to be at least a doubling of the number of doctors. Throughout the country, a closer marriage between teaching hospitals and the NHS was recommended. There was also a strong desire to improve relationships between hospitals, general practitioners and local authority services. The report's main emphasis however was on detailed guidance for the postgraduate period: vocational training in general practice and, for hospital staff, a period of general professional training in the main disciplines in approved posts. A section of the report dealt with the low quota of women admitted to medical schools arguing that there should be no gender bias; the criteria for admission should be the perceived ability of the candidate to profit from the course and become a good doctor.

The main proposals were acted on fairly quickly. Soon Higher Specialist Training Committees were established in the main branches of medicine, e.g. Medicine, Surgery, Psychiatry, Obstetrics and Gynaecology and the laboratory disciplines to advise on specialty training and approve the training posts throughout the country. Also the proportion of women entering the medical schools moved up to 50 per cent and sometimes more. Medical Schools' intake expanded to increase the output of doctors from around 2,000 per year to 4,000. A new medical school was being established in Nottingham and shortly there was to be another in Leicester.

Coincidentally at the end of the 1960s (1969-72) the Royal Colleges of Physicians finally agreed to a common MRCP examination, the MRCP (UK). London had always had a large entry for their examination and so did Edinburgh, which had a particularly high entry from the developing Commonwealth countries. This seemed to arise because very large numbers of overseas doctors had come to Edinburgh after the Second World War to take postgraduate courses and then go on to take the MRCP (Ed). What was new was that in Glasgow the Royal 'Faculty' had in the early 1960s become a Royal College of Physicians and Surgeons. Whereas the Faculty qualification attracted mainly local postgraduates, the College was now attracting increasing

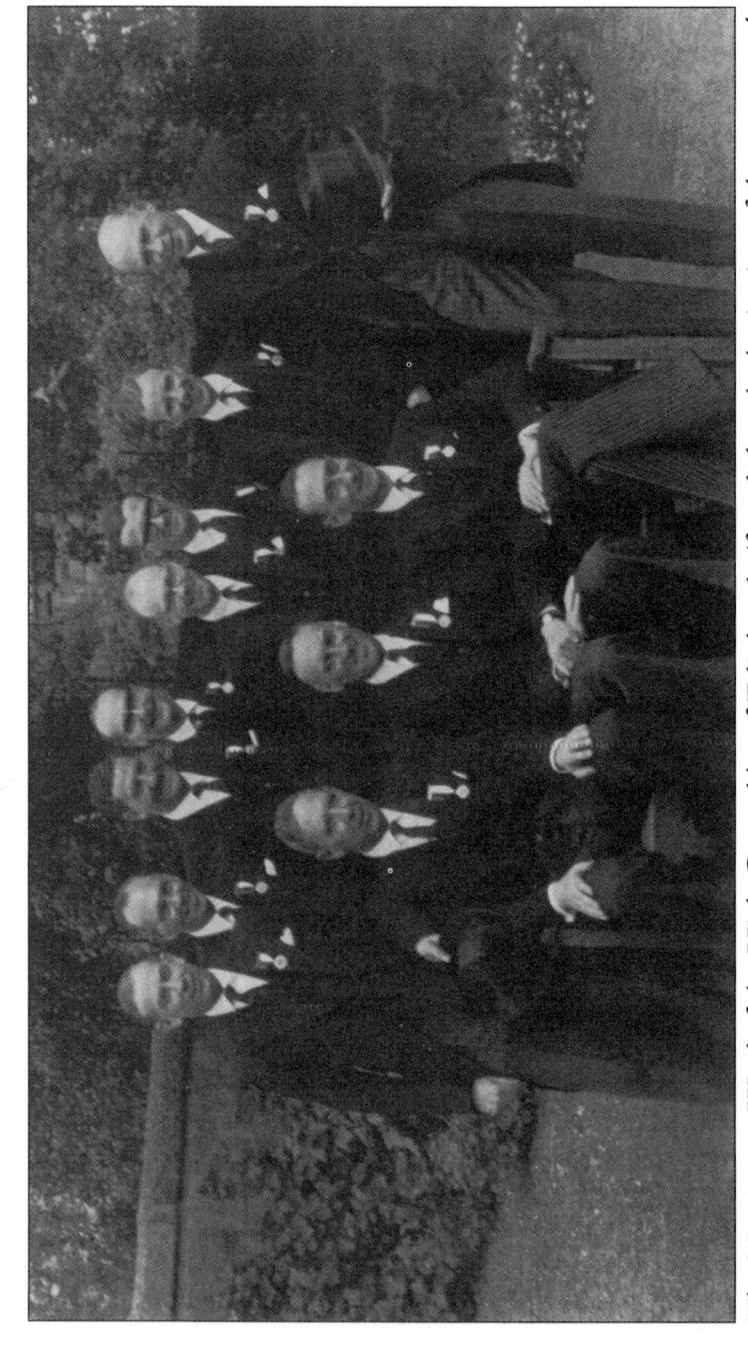

The Newington Ward of the High Constables of Edinburgh (founded at the beginning of the seventeenth century as the bodyguard of the Town Council). Richmond is third from the right in back row. My colleagues were all non-medical and represented a fascinating mixture of interests.

numbers from everywhere and its entry was approaching that of Edinburgh. We were moving into a strange position where many postgraduates, particularly from overseas were taking the Membership examination several times in all three UK Royal Colleges and some were also taking the examination in the Royal College of Physicians of Ireland in Dublin. The disease came to be known as 'multiple diplomatosis' and the introduction of the common MRCP (UK) examination could not have been more appropriate. Among other things this development was to lead to increasing symbiosis between the Royal Colleges over subsequent years, a happy development long overdue.

My time in Edinburgh certainly moulded my professional life and I was very comfortable with the mix of clinical work, teaching, examinations and research. I also had moved up from Senior Lectureship to Readership in the University. Perhaps, too early, I applied to succeed Sir Ian Hill in the Dundee Medical School but was unsuccessful. It seemed very likely that I would be staying in Edinburgh and there were lots of reasons for our accepting this as a good idea. Edinburgh was, and is, a lovely city. We had long-standing and happy friendships and these had been extended by all sorts of outside interests. I had for example been a High Constable of Edinburgh, an historical group originally committed to being the bodyguard of the Town Council but now paraded on ceremonial occasions. Number one son had started at Medical School in Edinburgh and number two son was about to start at Aberdeen. Our daughter was established in a good school and enjoying life. One particularly happy memory is our meeting with the first Captain of the first Polaris submarine which was refitting in Rosyth. We ended up having dinner on HMS *Resolution* at

Faslane and we have enjoyed keeping in touch with the Captain and his wife ever since.

However in the early 1970s there was no doubt that I was beginning to feel a little stale and during a spell when Professor Donald had sabbatical leave, I was given the role of Acting Head of the Department of Medicine. It was then that I realised that I would probably be happier running my own show.

CHAPTER 8

The 1970s and 1980s.
The Sheffield Medical School and the
Royal College of Physicians of London

THERE HAD BEEN TEACHING of Medicine in Sheffield for 150 years, at first as a College of the University of Manchester. Then in 1905 the Medical School became a Faculty within the University of Sheffield. The first full-time Professor of Medicine, Sir Charles Stuart-Harris was appointed in 1948 and his retirement in 1972 raised the possibility of an attractive move for me to pastures new.

However in the two or three weeks before the Appointments Committee was due to meet in the Spring of 1973, I had been invited to take part in a conference on the spleen in a small university town, Cluj in northern Rumania. Jenny accompanied me and we decided to go out by train, taking first the Orient Express from Ostend down the Rhine Valley for a stop off in Vienna. For the next stage of our journey we took the Simplon Orient Express which came down from Berlin. (There were several different Orient Expresses at the time.) At the Hungarian border there was a real 'iron curtain' with a large expanse of 'no-mans-land' and many sentry boxes high in the air. To our dismay we did not have visas to cross Hungary and were put off the train with our luggage down on the clinker as the train pulled out. I do not have great skills in foreign languages and certainly not in Hungarian and so it was unclear what was to happen.

Shortly we were put on a train going westwards back out to Austria, taken off at the first station, then whisked off in a high-speed car towards the Czechoslovakian border. I assumed that we were going to jail. However we were being taken to a car entry point where we were able to get visas. Then we were hurried back by car to the railway station and put on the next train out. We arrived in Budapest in the dark, late in the evening, in pouring rain and there was of course no chance of going further until next day.

For some strange reason a friend in Edinburgh had given me some Hungarian telephone tokens before departure and somehow I got the telephone number of the British Embassy. The voice said, 'Good evening, can I help you?' and I replied, 'Indeed you can.' We spent a good night in an Intercontinental Hotel across the square from the station and much of the next day in Budapest. The only remaining problem was that on reaching the Rumanian border there was a little further difficulty with the passports. Our visas had a car stamped on them and here we were travelling on a train and so where was our car? I think a nearby passenger with more linguistic skill than me was able to help us out.

Without much time to spare I was able to get back to Sheffield for the interview. I think that there was quite a robust contest for the appointment but I was fortunate to be successful.

Somehow Sheffield seemed to be a little isolated in people's memory. It used to be on the LMS railway line and most of the traffic going between south and north would travel on the east coast LNER line or on the A1. It was regarded as a dirty industrial city but if that was ever the case, it was no longer true. The heavy industry which had been in the van of the industrial revolution had been declining since the Second World War and accelerated by German bombs. In the early 1960s it had become the first 'clean air' city in the country. Moreover being contiguous with the Peak District of Derbyshire the environs were unexpectedly beautiful.

My own attraction to moving there, apart from wanting to head my own department, was the prospect of the medical school doubling in size, of the new hospital, the Hallamshire Hospital due to open shortly, and the plans to rebuild or restore or extend many of the district general hospitals, e.g. Barnsley, Doncaster, Chesterfield, Scunthorpe and further afield Grimsby and Hull in the surrounding areas. There was every indication of much enhancement of the medical services in this rather deprived part of the country.

In 1973 two old hospitals, the Royal Infirmary and the Royal Hospital were still the main loci for teaching near the University and they were to close and come together in the new Hallamshire Hospital.

I started in the Royal Hospital and could see from my room the new hospital on the nearby Beech Hill. Although it had won some award for architecture before the Second World War it was still a shell. I used to feel like Christian in *Pilgrim's Progress* looking over the 'slough of despond' to the 'celestial city'.

My first day had a few unusual happenings. The Outpatient Department of the Royal Hospital had been based in an old chapel but was now translocated to the ground floor of the unfinished Hallamshire Hospital. I got out of my car in the early morning and an old consultant said in Yorkshire dialect, 'A new face. Who are you?' I said, rejoicing in my new title, 'I am Professor Richmond,' to which he responded, 'Oh, and what do you profess?' I said

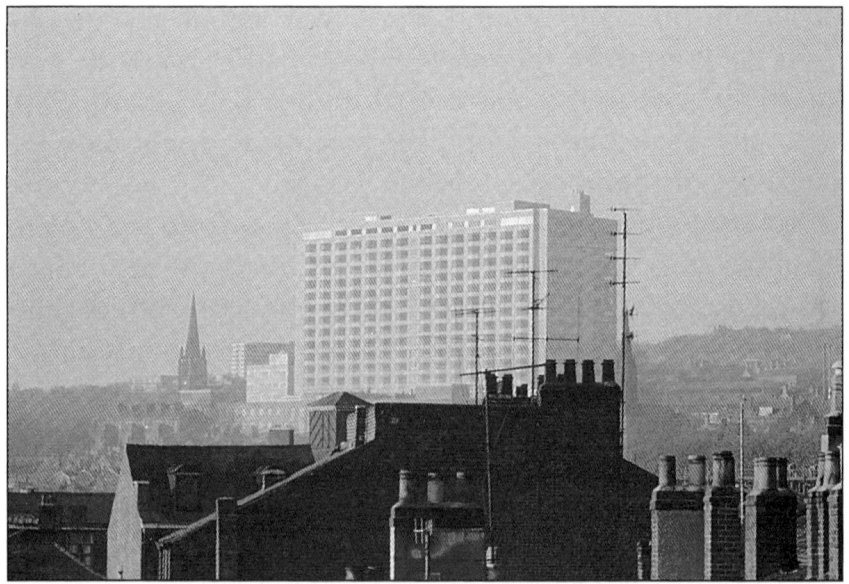

The (Royal) Hallamshire Hospital, Sheffield. For five years the Professor of Medicine looks out of his room at the still unfinished new hospital rather like Christian in Pilgrim's Progress looking at the Celestial City over the Slough of Despond.

that I was the Professor of Medicine which drew the surprising remark, 'Oh, you'll get some grand experience here; stand you in very good stead when you're applying for your next job!' And that was my first five minutes in my new job.

That evening there was a nice reception for the new fellow and I noticed that many of the senior people were Scottish – and here was I coming from Edinburgh. I went over to ingratiate myself with one of the old Sheffield physicians and got round to saying that I had been born in England. He wanted to know where and I told him Doncaster. I got another unexpected remark, 'My goodness, Richmond, if I was you I would keep that to yourself!'

But the other memory of the first day during which my unit was receiving emergency admissions was that I saw some very strange medical problems. One was a teenage boy who had profound anaemia but had been working on a farm until the previous day; it emerged that his bowels had not moved for six weeks, eight weeks or even more. I am happy to record that in due course all was well. Another was a middle-aged man, very confused and disabled. He had striking pinpoint pupils of the eyes not reacting to light but reacting to accommodation. These were so-called Argyll Robertson pupils. I had not seen these landmarks of third-stage syphilis for many years, nor had the consultant who specialised in sexually transmitted disease. The patient was of course suffering from 'general paralysis of the insane'. I have not met that diagnosis again.

After some five years the Hallamshire Hospital was ready for occupation and later it was made Royal by HRH the Prince of Wales. A recollection of the move from the Royal Hospital was that in lifting piles of books into boxes in my room I got an acute prolapse of a lumbar intervertebral disc. This required fairly urgent surgery, a laminectomy, but this was enormously successful because I was able to dive off rocks in the Mediterranean only four weeks later!

I was in hospital for only a few days but the Minister of my (Presbyterian) church came to see me once or twice. One day, as he was arriving, a senior nun, who had been a patient of mine for some time, was leaving my room. My Minister said, 'I see that you are keeping your options open!'

Most specialties were represented in the new hospital, the Children's Hospital, the Women's Hospital, the Radio-therapy Hospital and the Dental School being nearby but separate. The Professorial Medical Unit occupied two of the seven medical wards and therefore catered for two-sevenths of the medical elective and emergency admissions.

The hospital was delightful with bright four-bedded wards and each unit had four single rooms at either end, which were ideal for those patients needing privacy or isolation. The four-bedded wards had large south-facing windows and at first we encouraged 'open' visiting. The 'open' visiting soon had to be curtailed however because visitors sometimes came with their sandwiches to sit at the windows all day admiring the view!

I had inherited from Sir Charles Stuart-Harris very strong sections of respiratory medicine and renal medicine, the former having an international research reputation in respiratory physiology. Shortly we were to add a special interest in liver disease.

Haematology was already well represented in Sheffield and in any case my own active research days were winding down. The main commitment was to encourage research and fund-raising in others. Radiotherapy was very well represented also but significantly chemotherapy was now emerging as a very critical part of cancer care. My past interest in oncology was helpful. Much has happened since then but in the early 1970s it became possible with new chemotherapy regimes to bring malignant disease of the lymphatic system (Hodgkin's disease and non-Hodgkin's lymphoma) and some leukaemias under control and cures were beginning to emerge. One young lady that I particularly remember from the early days had advanced Hodgkin's disease and would normally have been expected to succumb in less than eighteen months. She was still alive and well when last I heard, twenty-five years later.

The evolution of clinical oncology in collaboration with

the Radiotherapy Hospital was greatly prospered by the generosity of the Yorkshire Cancer Research Campaign. In due course we were able to establish an academic department with professorial head and this now is highly regarded on the national stage.

The increase in student numbers from around eighty entrants per year to 160 soon got under way. One new departure was to output most of them for a few weeks during their clinical years to the district general hospitals. Not only did this extend their experience but also a consequence was that many of them went back to these hospitals to do their first posts on graduating and this improved these hospitals' junior staffing numbers which could sometimes be difficult to maintain. As the central hospitals in Sheffield were developing so was the large Northern General Hospital in the northern part of the city and the facilities for all the essential components of a Medical School were reaching levels of excellence. The Northern General Hospital from the early 1970s had been adding academic departments with professorial heads and my opposite number and partner in medicine was Professor Donald Munro. Whereas the Trent Region of England, with a population of 5 million like that of Scotland, had been the most deprived in England in the early years of the National Health Service, this was no longer so. Also Sheffield had had the only University and Medical School in the Region. There was now one in Nottingham and another evolving in Leicester.

Again one is reminded of our very small world. One particularly happy friendship was with the Regional Medical Officer, the late Professor James Scott, who had been in his first year at Doncaster Grammar School when I had been in my last.

Overseas visits were becoming a stimulating part of life. In the 1970s I had two trips to Khartoum in Sudan, an interesting city at the junction of the White Nile and the Blue Nile where, in the Medical School, there was a long British tradition. My host, the Professor of Medicine, had been in Edinburgh in the 1960s for postgraduate experience and the MRCP (Ed) examination. Iraq also had a long British tradition and Medical City, the medical school component of the University of Baghdad, had had many British teachers. On my first visit there for one month, Jenny accompanied me and we stayed in the Baghdad Hotel on the banks of the River Tigris. On arrival at the airport, a doctor was seeing off a visitor and he also had passed through Edinburgh in the 1960s. He and his wife overwhelmed us with kindness during our stay. By the time of the second visit, a few years later, there had been many developments, particularly of modern hotels, I believe for an expected visit of the Organisation of African Unity. This time I stayed in the Mansour Melia Hotel on the other side of the river. Unfortunately the Iran/Iraq war had started although at the time activity was mainly in the south in the Basra area. However occasional bombs were dropping in Baghdad. The most alarming experience occurred one day when I had gone on a trip to Babylon. Apparently in the morning a group of Iranian fanatics had driven a bus full of explosives into the radio station across the road from the Mansour Melia. When I returned, the side of my hotel had been blown in and if I had been in my room, I would not be here today. I may say that it put one off having an evening stroll! Around this time there were also visits either for teaching or to take part in examinations to Ibadan in Nigeria and Kuala Lumpur in Malaysia.

I was still being active in MRCP (UK) examinations, often in Edinburgh but was now in some of those based in London. In the late 1970s the London College held a Regional Conference in Sheffield and on the last evening Jenny and I had a little gathering at home for some colleagues and the College visitors. The London-based MRCP (UK), apart from some extramural examinations during the Second World War, was always held in London. The clinical examinations were conducted in the London hospitals in the mornings and then the candidates and examiners repaired to the College in Regent's Park for oral examinations in the afternoons. I should explain that the MRCP (UK) then comprised a multiple-choice paper as Part I of the examination and if successful the candidates who were allowed only a limited number of attempts could proceed to Part II, but within the next five years. Part II had a written part after which if successful, the candidate could go on some six weeks later to the clinical and oral examination. Again only a limited number of attempts were permitted.

I remember, perhaps impertinently, suggesting to the visitors that it would be splendid if places like Sheffield could occasionally host the examination (the clinical and oral part). I learned that on the train on the way back to London this was discussed and provisionally approved. Shortly Sheffield was to host a wing of the examination on five consecutive occasions to get the provisional 'bugs' out of it and it is now regularly held in centres all over the country.

There are often amusing episodes during examinations and perhaps I may recount one from Sheffield. In the clinical examination there used to be one 'long case' which tested history taking and physical examination and also multiple 'quickies' on short cases. There would perhaps be five to six short cases or more, patients who kindly helped us so that various bodily systems could be tested. We had a porter in the Royal Hallamshire Hospital who had a rare but often used problem, 'dystrophia myotonica'. This disorder has several components including slow relaxation of grip but can usually be spotted because of frontal baldness, droopy eyelids and some wasting of facial muscles. My porter would sometimes stand in and help me if we needed more short cases. One day I was introducing a candidate to my porter and he obviously had no idea what he was observing. Trying to be helpful I suggested to the candidate that he might speak to the porter. He said, 'Tell me, sir, what is troubling you?' to which the porter responded, 'I've got dystrophia myotonica.' Needless to say we had to move on to the next patient without further ado.

I had been on the Council of the College which is by election but was soon a Pro-Censor and then a Censor. However the greatest honour of all came in 1984-5 when I became Senior Censor and Senior Vice-President which I have to confess was then by invitation. Then followed Chairmanship of the MRCP (UK) part II Examining Board (1985-9), an excellent period for helping to cement good ties between London, Glasgow and Edinburgh.

Overseas visits now seemed to accelerate and Jenny was able to join me on several of them. There were visits to the medical school in Kuwait and to a new school in the Eastern Province of Saudi Arabia, in King Faisal University near Dammam and Dahran. On one of my visits to Saudi Arabia I woke one morning in my hotel room to find that the English version of the *Arab Times* had been pushed under my door. I glanced through it cursorily but did notice on the sports page at the back a curious heading in large letters: 'Big Jack leaves Wednesday'. This did not ring any bells, but in the evening I realised that Jack Charlton was leaving Sheffield Wednesday. Obviously the local people knew more about English football than I did!

In Saudi Arabia, where I went several times, the separation of the women from the men was particularly evident. The women were academically excellent and in the hospital their clinical teaching and the examinations seemed to present no difficulty. I do recall one incident however which I hope does not cause offence. I usually would shake hands with a candidate before embarking on a clinical examination hoping to put him/her at their ease. One young woman said, 'I am very sorry but I am not allowed to shake hands with a man,' but shortly she was examining a man's bare abdomen as an essential part of my assessment. The Professor of Medicine who was paired with me and whom I have seen in recent years still has a little chuckle over the episode.

I have often recounted another episode with a woman student and this was also during an undergraduate examination in Dublin. The medical school was based on the Royal College of Surgeons and on a particular morning I had to be off early to do the clinical examination at Drogheda. The very first candidate was a most stunning looking girl and I was thinking privately that she might not have had much time to concentrate on her medical studies. However as soon as we got started it was clear that she was outstanding and as we went on she got better and better and realised that she was doing well. Then we had to return to Dublin for the oral examinations in the afternoon. The woman had an 'Honours' oral with other examiners. The

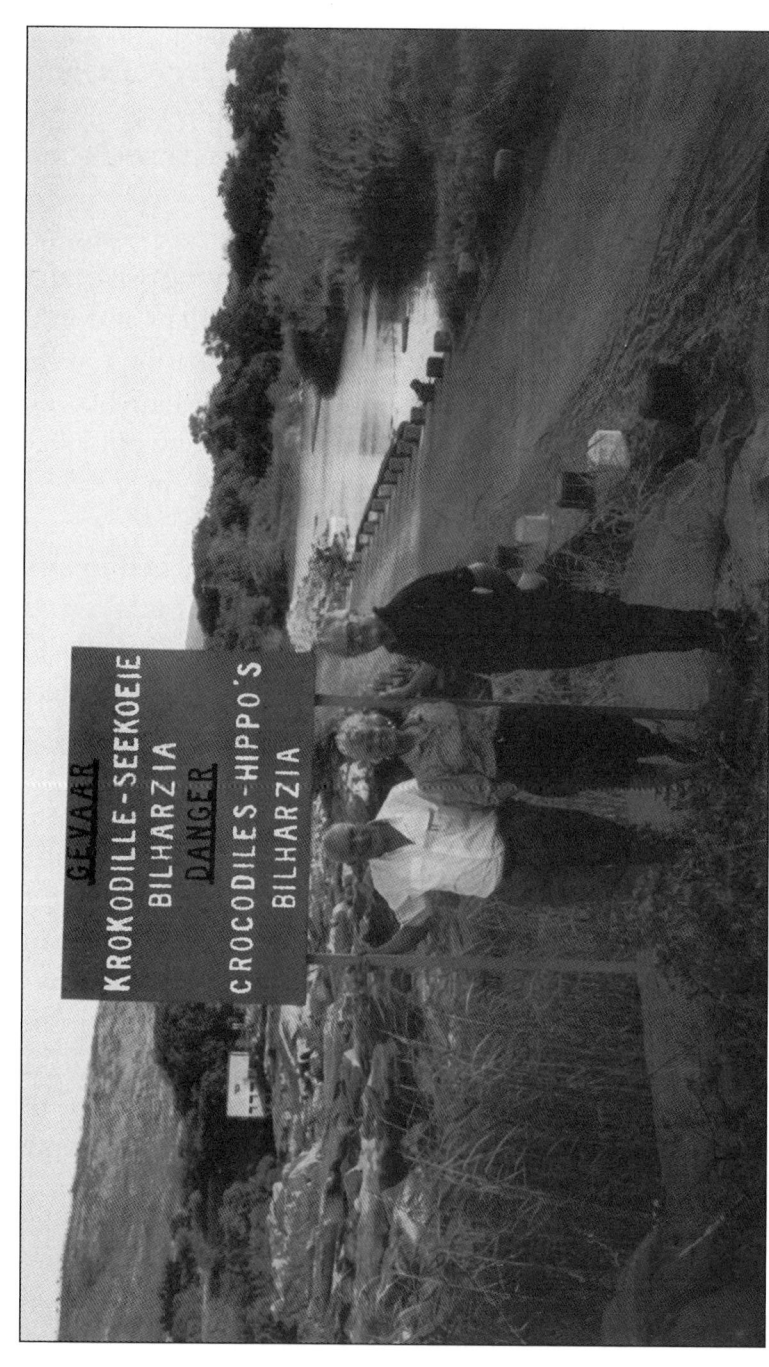

On the Crocodile River at Nelspruit near the Mozambique border with Dr George Campbell. Bilharzia is a human disease caught from snails.

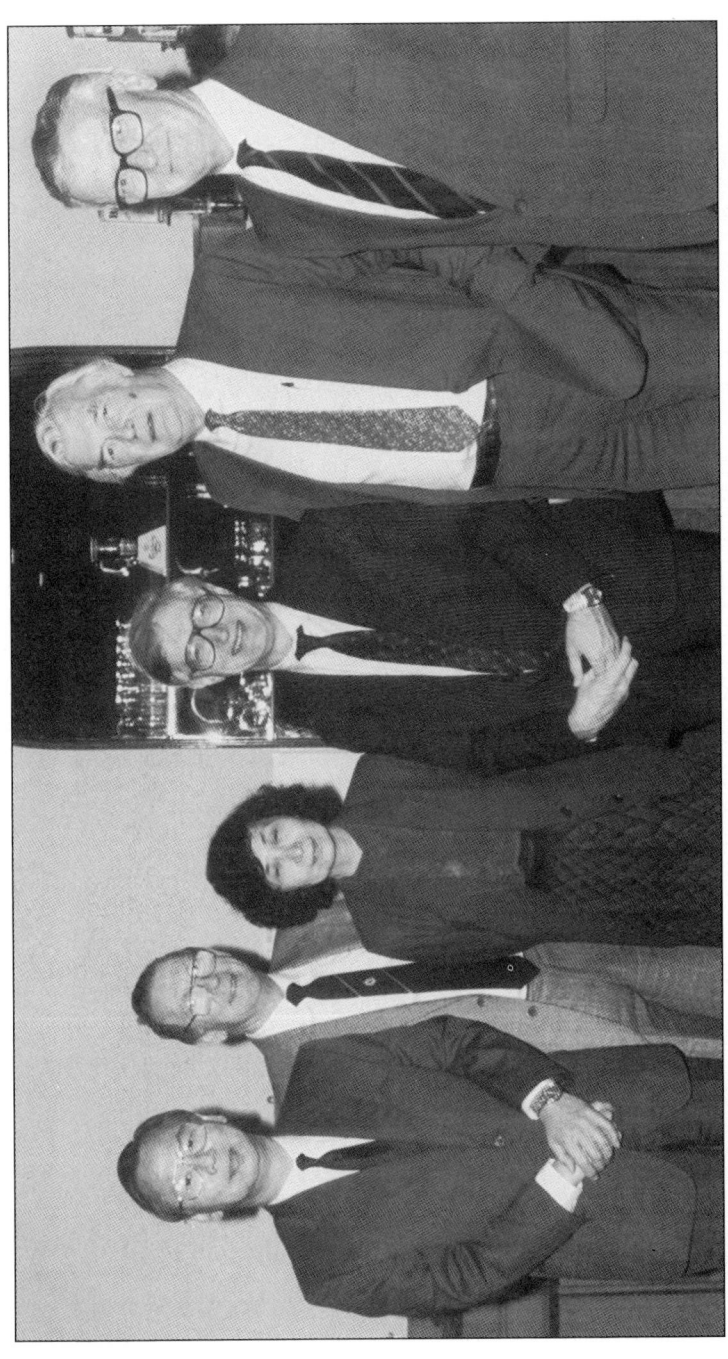

Hong Kong, 1987. With the examiners for the clinical and oral examinations of the MRCP (UK) Part II. Professor David Todd is on the left and Professor Vallance-Owen, second from right, the two Professors of Medicine in Hong Kong at the time.

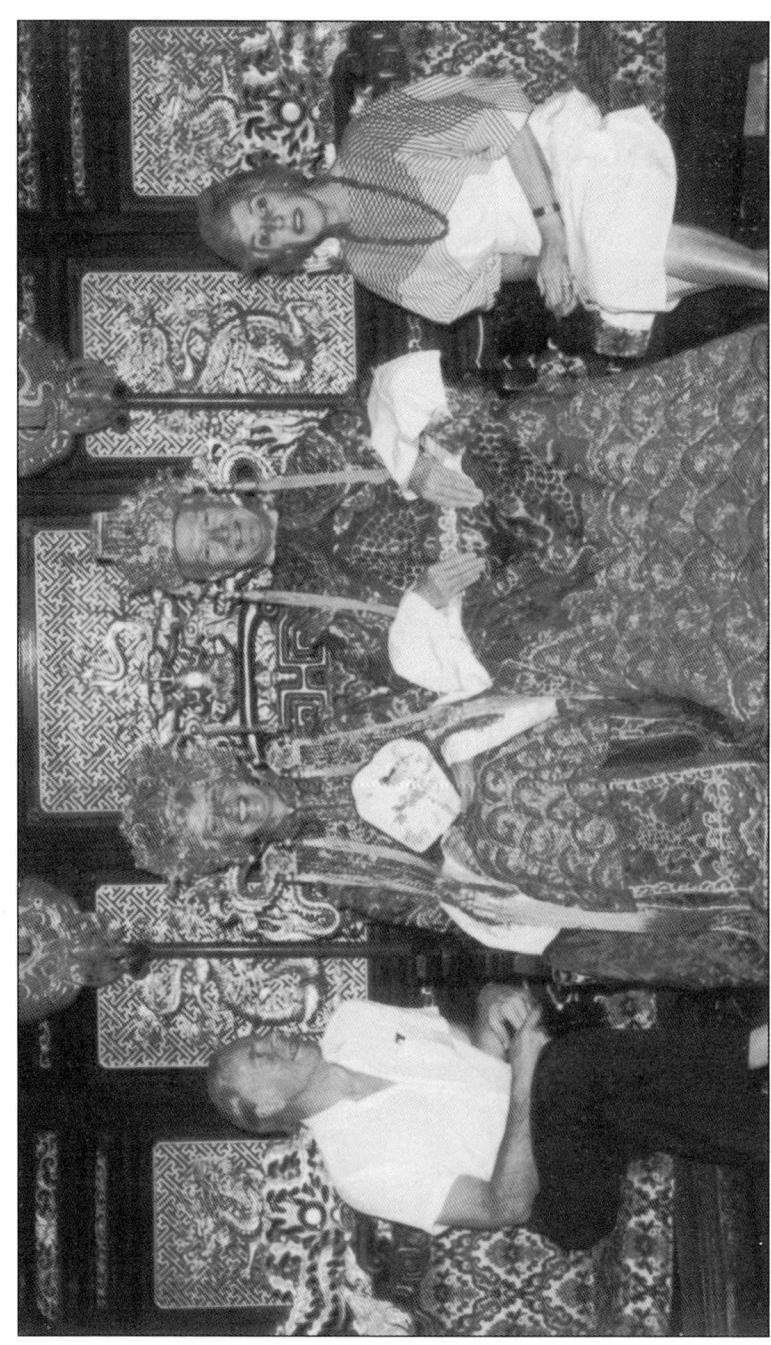

Jenny and me installed as 'King and Queen' at the Jumbo Floating Restaurant, Hong Kong. Professor and Mrs Michael Oliver are with us, 1987.

long day's work was over by about 6 p.m. and I was feeling somewhat weary. However our hosts wanted us to have a little session in a pub behind the College. The place was dark and filled with smoke and out of the gloom appeared my woman candidate. Before I fully recognised her she gave me an enormous kiss and thanked me for being 'such a pet'!

I had around this time two examining visits to the Medical School in Harare, Zimbabwe where Professor Jimmy Thomas was now in charge. There were return visits to Malaysia but most emphasis was now in Singapore where they were developing a sophisticated postgraduate examination, the M. Med. In Malaysia and Singapore most of the physician teachers were Fellows of one or more of the UK colleges. Many M. Med candidates would follow their local examination by travelling to the UK to attempt the MRCP (UK).

The Part I of the MRCP (UK) had been held in many overseas centres for several years. Then, for the first time, the clinical and oral examinations of the Part II were exported to Hong Kong. I much enjoyed taking part in the early visits in 1985-8 both to examinations in the University of Hong Kong on the Island and in the new Chinese University at Shatin in the New Territories. Now the Part II examination is being held in several overseas centres.

In 1985-8 I was Dean of Medicine and Dentistry in Sheffield, a commitment that tended to come by rote. It was quite an onerous period because at that time severe financial constraints were being applied to Universities and saving monies in a Medical School, particularly on staffing, is not easy. However retirement was looming and I was already, with Jenny, beginning to think of our returning to our spiritual home in Edinburgh.

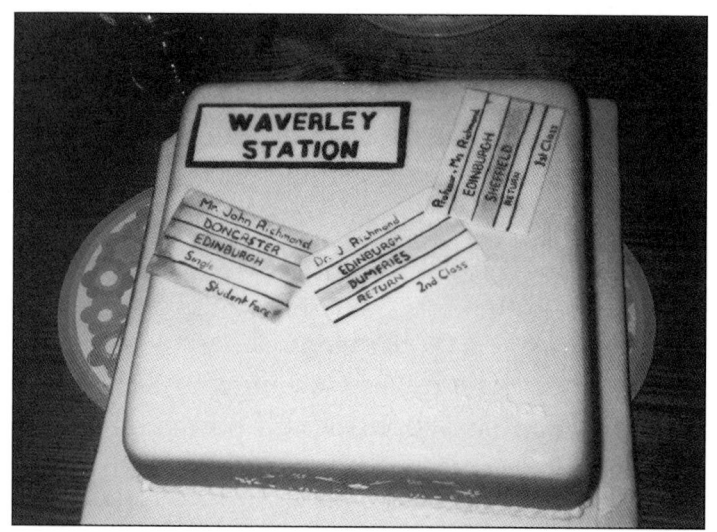

A farewell cake with 'All good wishes' prepared for me by the technicians in my Department of Medicine in Sheffield.

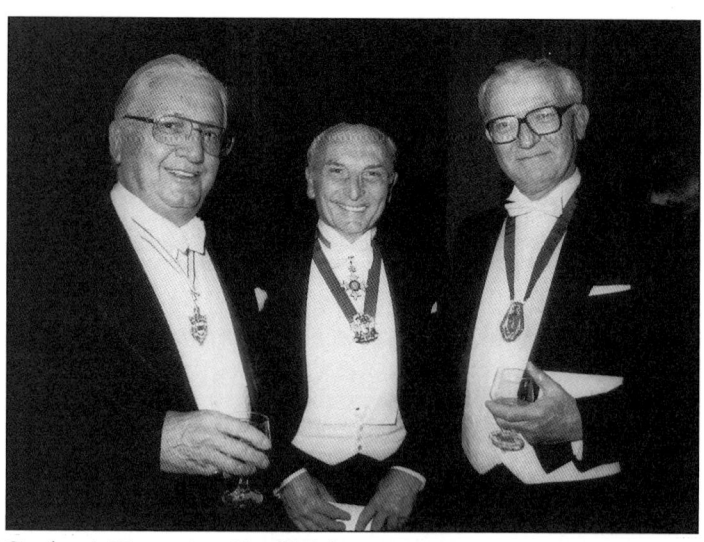

The Cutlers' Feast in Sheffield in 1989. On the left is Mr Peter McGhie, a Past Master of the Company. In the middle is Sir Peter Heatley, at the time Master of the Merchant Company in Edinburgh. Sir Peter preceded me as Edinburgh University Diving Champion.

Before I move on from Sheffield I have to record how good and rewarding was the interdisciplinary and inter-Faculty mixing that there was in the University. But more than that we seemed to meet many people socially outside medicine and very many are continuing good friends. One great and lasting memory was to be asked to propose the toast to the historic Cutlers' Company of Sheffield at their annual Cutlers' Feast. It was of course a delightful and unforgettable occasion.

CHAPTER 9

Presidency of the Royal College of Physicians of Edinburgh, 1988-91

UNTIL 1950 IT WAS NOT possible to be considered for election to the Council of the Royal College of Physicians of Edinburgh unless one was domiciled within 'septem millia' (7 miles) of the General Post Office. When this law was expunged in 1950 a more nationwide representation could be considered. I had of course kept many ties with Edinburgh alive with frequent visits for University and College examinations and it seems to have been known that Richmond and his wife were planning to return to 'Auld Reekie'. And so it was that at the end of 1987 it was suggested that I might like my name to go forward for election to the Council and I was delighted to agree. When retiring from an active and busy professional life it can be disastrous to pull the shutters down and to ossify; this was going to be an excellent way of winding down gradually and reviving many old friendships and happy memories.

Election to the Council followed and then one year later, election to the Presidency. I was the 121st President (since 1681) but because of the earlier geographical restrictions, I was only the third from outside Edinburgh and the first from residence in England. The first was Professor, later Sir Ian Hill, from Dundee in 1963, my first physician chief, and the second was Dr Christopher Clayson from Lochmaben in Dumfriesshire in 1966.

These movements from the Medical School in Edinburgh to the Medical School in Sheffield and then having been in a senior position in the London College, transferring allegiance to the Edinburgh College, have led to one or two slightly hurtful comments. An erstwhile colleague in Scotland has termed me a 'carpetbagger'. Also not long ago, in London, I was referred to as 'that renegade Scot'! If that is what people think, so be it. I look back on my life and could feel embarrassed that it was so totally unplanned. What happens is that doors open and one senses that there could be great excitement beyond.

For the first year I continued as Professor of Medicine in Sheffield but this was not very fair to Sheffield or to Edinburgh because the Presidency was becoming a fairly full-time job. There is an excellent President's flat in the College and I stayed there over many nights but sometimes would return to Sheffield late at night by car after dinner if I had some important commitment e.g. teaching, next day. It seemed sensible to retire from Sheffield a little early and this I did in Autumn 1989. One of these nocturnal journeys is remembered with particular clarity. When getting near Scotch Corner, I realised that I had left the key of our Sheffield house in a jacket pocket back in the College. We phoned neighbours who had a key and got no reply. Then we phoned number two son, who was now a consultant in Sheffield, and daughter-in-law because they were taking over our house and also had a key, only to discover that they had lost it. We arrived in Sheffield at 2.30 a.m. in pouring rain. All the downstairs windows were double glazed and so entry had to be sought through an upstairs window. We had an appropriate ladder and, as I have mentioned earlier, despite my high-board diving career I feel dizzy if I am more than a few feet above ground. And so, to my shame, the redoubtable Jenny had to break in through the bathroom window upstairs and get in!

Medical practice in Scotland goes back for many centuries and it is of interest to rehearse a little of the early history. I am indebted to the President and Council of the Edinburgh College for allowing me to access *The History of The Royal College of Physicians of Edinburgh* by W.S. Craig for some of what follows.

The first move to any organisation would be the establishment of the Institute of Surgeons and Barber Surgeons in Edinburgh mentioned in Chapter 3 which received its Royal Seal of Cause from James IV in 1505. It is of course now the Royal College of Surgeons of Edinburgh.

In the 1600s most non-surgical problems were dealt with by the 'Apothecaries' but there was increasing need to regulate medical as opposed to surgical practice. Important observations were being made and perhaps the one that had particular impact was the great William Harvey's description of the circulation of the blood in his treatise 'De motu cardis' in 1628.

There is one fascinating story from around this time which is not widely known. When James VI went down to London in 1603 to inherit the English throne after the death of Elizabeth I, he took with him his physician, John Craig. The physicians of the London College (established in Henry VIII's time) kicked up a fuss because Craig was a foreigner but James was having no nonsense and naturalised him on the spot. Some months later, when a vacancy occurred Craig was examined and admitted to Fellowship of the London College. On the same day an Englishman was examined for the second time and then twice more over several months before being received into Fellowship. The Englishman was William Harvey!

Moves to establish a College of Physicians in Edinburgh had started around the same time but had foundered when James VI moved to England. Strangely, it was in Cromwell's time as Lord Protector that a Charter emerged contemplating the establishment in Edinburgh of a College of Physicians for Scotland. This had developed through submission to Cromwell and his Lords of Council of a list of 'Publik Abuses' and these in detail make absorbing reading. The list included 'frequent murders' by quacks and others; the 'unlimited practices' by surgeons and apothecaries without advice from physicians; the unlimited 'vending' and 'exorbitant' prices of drugs; the great expense and difficulty for students seeking medical education and degrees which could only be obtained abroad; and the great loss to physicians who could not improve their learning with the aid of professors.

Naturally there was enormous opposition to a proposed College of Physicians of Scotland from the Surgeons, the Glasgow Faculty (established in 1599), the apothecaries, Edinburgh Town Council, Scottish Universities other than Edinburgh that had been awarding occasional medical degrees without formal education, and surprisingly, the Church. The prime movers among the physicians in Edinburgh were Dr George Sibbald and later Dr George Purves, but eventually Sir Robert Sibbald (George Sibbald's nephew) succeeded in establishing the Royal College of Physicians of Edinburgh, the Royal charter being awarded by Charles II in November 1681.

A measure of protection was provided for the Physicians by the Charter decreeing that the Surgeons 'shall by no means have the care of diseases originally internal, solely to be undertaken by the prescription and direction of Physicians of the said College'. One interesting corollary was that Obstetrics was considered as something originally internal and was therefore in the province of the Physicians. Indeed Sir James Young Simpson, the discoverer of chloroform, Professor of Midwifery in the University of Edinburgh, became President of the College as late as 1850-2. The Faculty of Physicians and Surgeons in Glasgow was understandably reassured when the new College was to be defined as of Edinburgh, and not of Scotland.

And so in 1681 Sir Robert Sibbald along with twenty other founding Fellows set about the task of making the practice of medicine a reputable science, alleviating the miseries of the sick and the poor and putting the prescription and the use of drugs on a proper footing. In the early years (1699) the Fellows published the Edinburgh Pharmacopoeia which received much acclaim and it was not until some twelve further editions that it was superseded in 1864 by the British Pharmacopoeia.

Also the College began to award after examination its licence to practise medicine. Now the College's examination MRCP (UK) is not a licence to initiate practice but a critical evaluation of postgraduate progress leading to membership of all the UK colleges, election to Fellowship of one or more of the colleges following a few years later after a period of distinguished professional service. The Colleges of Physicians' primary objective is to maintain and pursue the highest standards in medicine.

By the terms of the 1681 Charter the College was not permitted to provide teaching courses but many of the Fellows, particularly those who had received their primary training from Boerhaave in Leiden, Holland (see Chapter 3) were to become teachers in Edinburgh University's Faculty of Medicine when it was founded in 1726.

In the early days the founding Fellows of the College would meet in each other's houses and then in small meeting rooms because it was not until 1704 that the first college building was established. This was in Fountain Close in the old town of Edinburgh off the Royal Mile. The Old Town was then a relatively small community domiciled mainly along and near the ridge extending from the Castle, to the great rock, Arthur's Seat. The next College, a splendid but apparently unsuitable building was in the New Town at the east end of George Street. The magnificent New Town, that part of Edinburgh northwards from the Castle, was envisioned and largely planned by James Craig.

The new College, our present one, was built in 1844-6 at the east end of the parallel Queen Street. What is now the central building and embracing the 'Great Hall' was designed by the architect Thomas Hamilton. In 1864, the house on the east side, the very first house in Queen Street, built in 1770-2, and designed by the famous Robert Adam for the Lord Chief Baron Orde of the Scottish Court of the Exchequer, was purchased by the College. In the 1980s the house on the other side was acquired and converted into a magnificent Conference Centre. More recently further adjoining properties have been added to embrace the College's burgeoning activities and influence.

The foregoing is a summary of the marvellous heritage which it was a great honour to serve albeit briefly. Apart from the history already alluded to, the long list of past

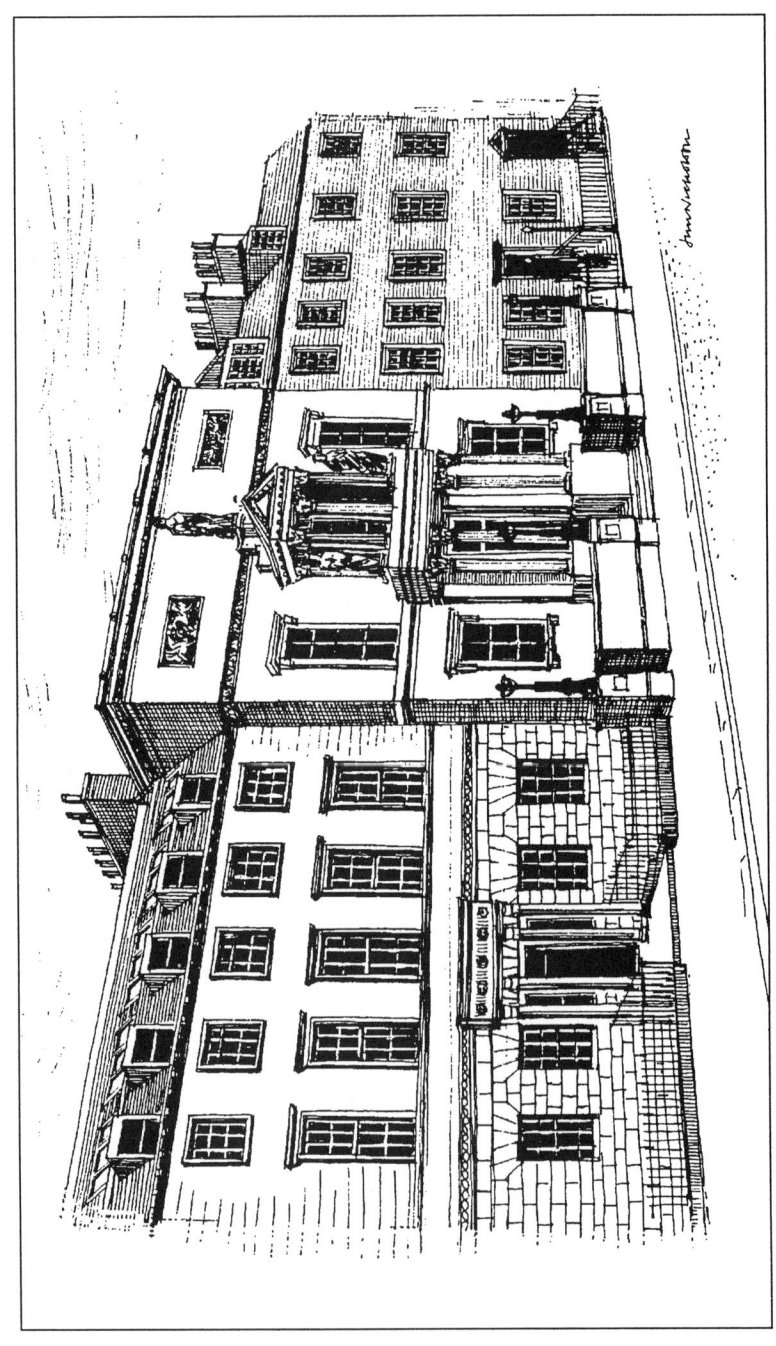

Royal College of Physicians, Edinburgh with Great Hall Building in the centre, Robert Adam House to the left and Conference Centre to the right.

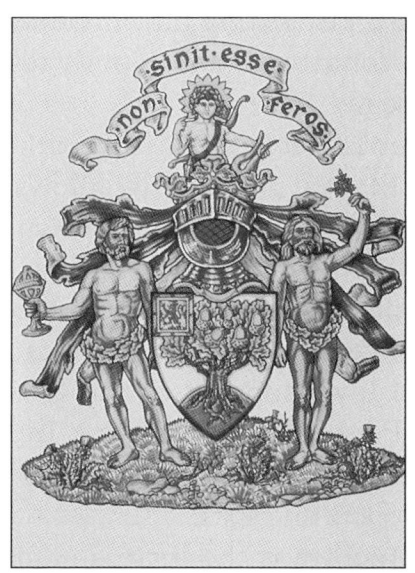

Crest of Royal College of Physicians of Edinburgh. It was unusual to have the shield held by two savages and to include the Lion of Scotland.

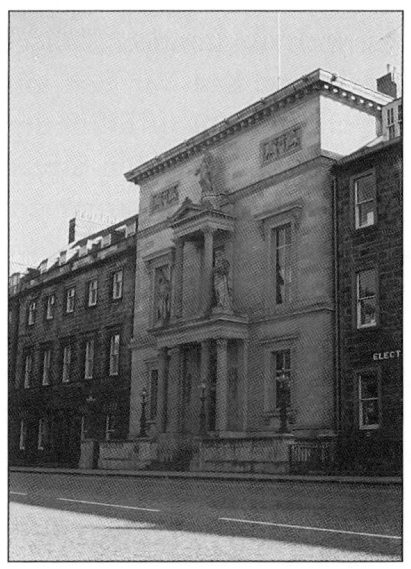

Royal College of Physicians of Edinburgh in Queen Street with Robert Adam House beyond.

presidents is also fascinating and includes many of great distinction who contributed enormously to the teaching and practice of medicine.

The President is elected annually at the time of the St Andrew's Day Festival and usually allows his name to go forward for a second and third year. And so it was that I was in office from 1988-91. It is difficult to reflect on all the things that happened during that period because so much has happened since. In any case nothing is possible without the selfless and loyal support of the Council then quite small, the Vice-President, the Secretary, Treasurer, Librarian, Editor of College publications, the College Manager and all their excellent supporting staff.

One development was the increasing desire of the UK Colleges to come together and meet formally more with each other. We had of course many contacts through various national committees. However we had our first joint scientific symposia with the London College for 300 years. I was boasting also that we had our first joint meeting with the Royal College of Surgeons of Edinburgh which is sited less than one mile away from Queen Street, only to be told by Miss Ferguson, our then Librarian, to whom I owe a great deal, that I had made a mistake – we had a meeting with the surgeons in the 1830s. The animosity between the physicians and the surgeons to which I have already referred continued for a very long time. Now we cannot live without each other. Happily the Colleges of Physicians and Surgeons, including the ones in Dublin and the many specialist Colleges and Faculties based in London are gradually joining together as a collaborating family.

A feature of the Edinburgh College of Physicians has long been the large proportion of its Fellowship based overseas, mainly in the Commonwealth. Usually during a President's term of office there will be a formal visit and conference with a college in a far away country. In 1988 when I was on the Council, we had an excellent meeting in Singapore. In my time the main event was a joint meeting with the College of Physicians and Surgeons of Pakistan. This was in September 1990 and there were some misgivings about proceeding with the plan because Benazir Bhutto had recently been deposed and the country was in a state of emergency. However I am glad that we went ahead because all went well and our hosts had made enormously generous preparation for our visit. Quite a large group of Fellows with many wives made the trip.

The Pakistan College, then thirty years old, was based in Karachi and we started there. First there was a Convocation when honours were bestowed and exchanged, then there was a scientific meeting, the visit to Karachi ending with a splendid banquet. Then we separated into two groups, one going to Multan and Lahore with the Vice-President, Dr Tony Toft, and my group going to Peshawar and Islamabad where the two groups would meet up. At each place we had joint scientific meetings. At Peshawar it was essential that we traversed the Khyber Pass through the Tribal Territories to the Afghanistan border. Not only did we have a military escort but also we were comforted to be shown military groups in the hills ensuring our safety. One interesting piece of information was that some 90 per cent of the established physicians in the North West Frontier Province of Pakistan were Fellows of the Edinburgh College. In Islamabad the Minister of Health, also an FRCP (Ed) met us all for our final gathering. Several of the Fellows asked me to convey greetings to landladies in Edinburgh of whom they spoke

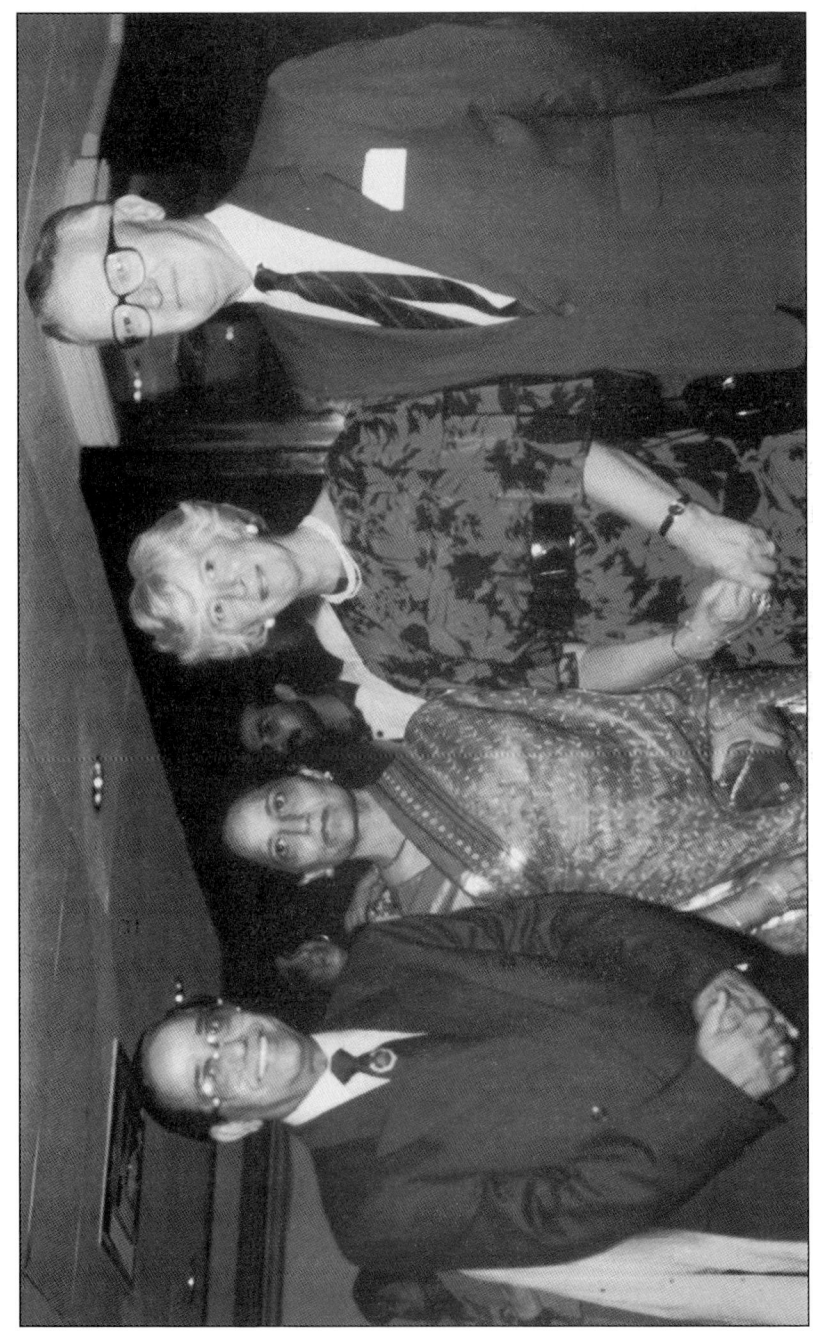

Jenny and me with Professor and Mrs Rab, Pakistan.

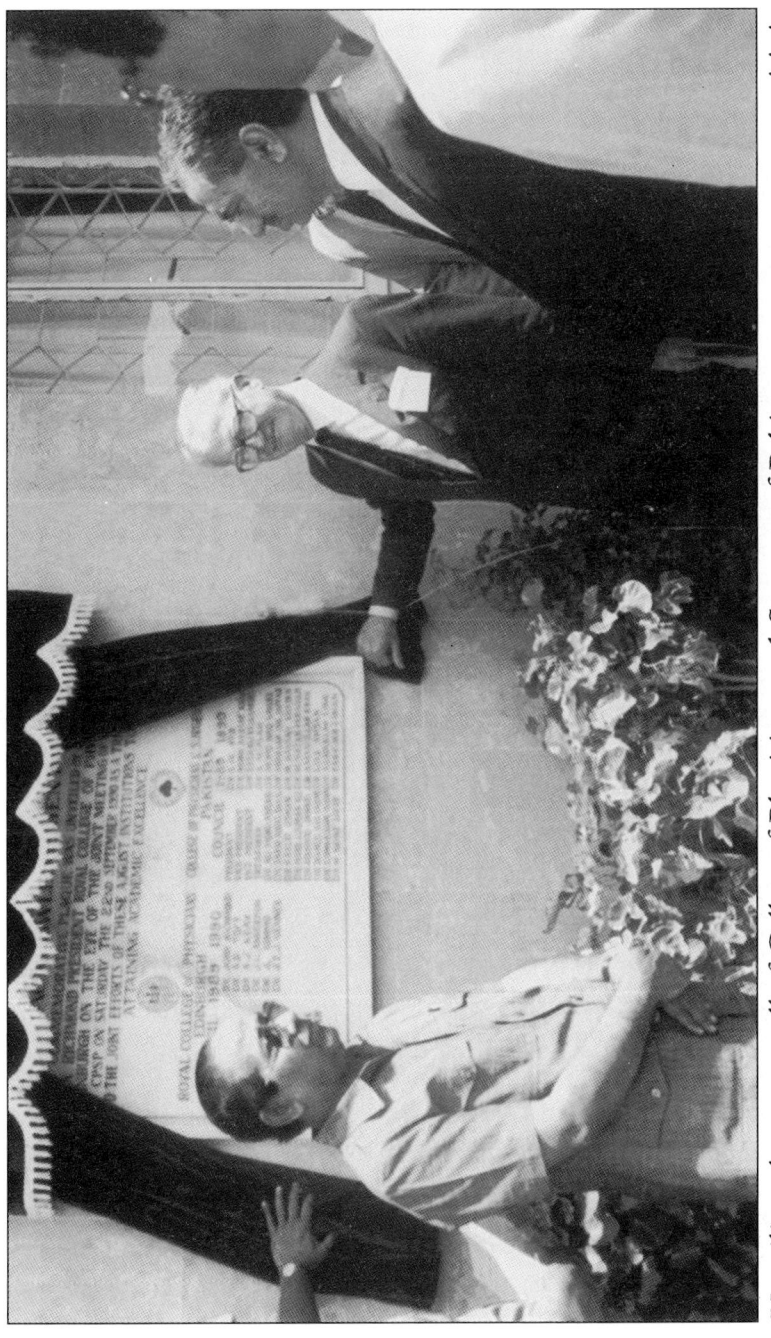

Unveiling plaque on wall of College of Physicians and Surgeons of Pakistan to commemorate our visit in September 1990. Minister of Health on the right and Professor S.M. Rab, President of College on the left.

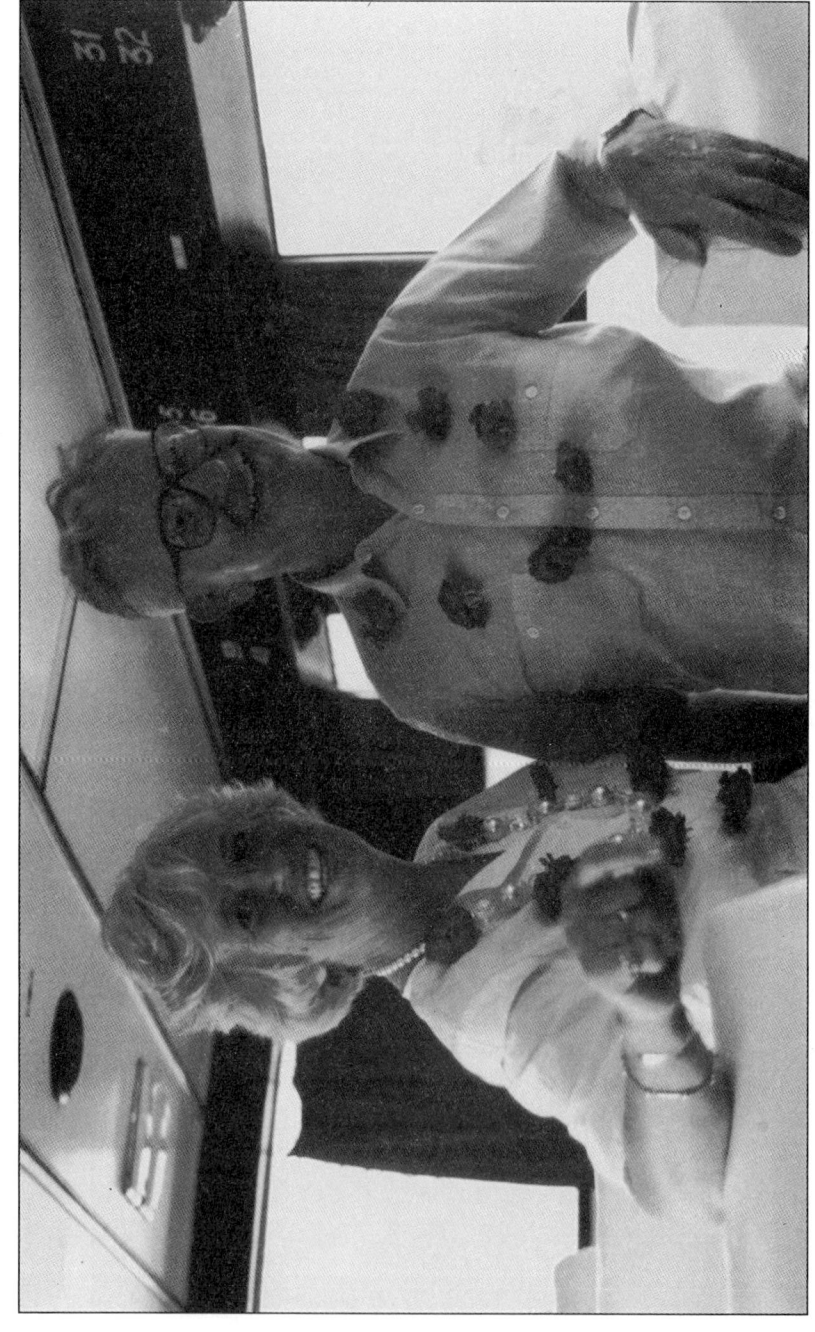

Jenny and I on sightseeing bus tour of Karachi. This was much enjoyed and we are garlanded as the guests.

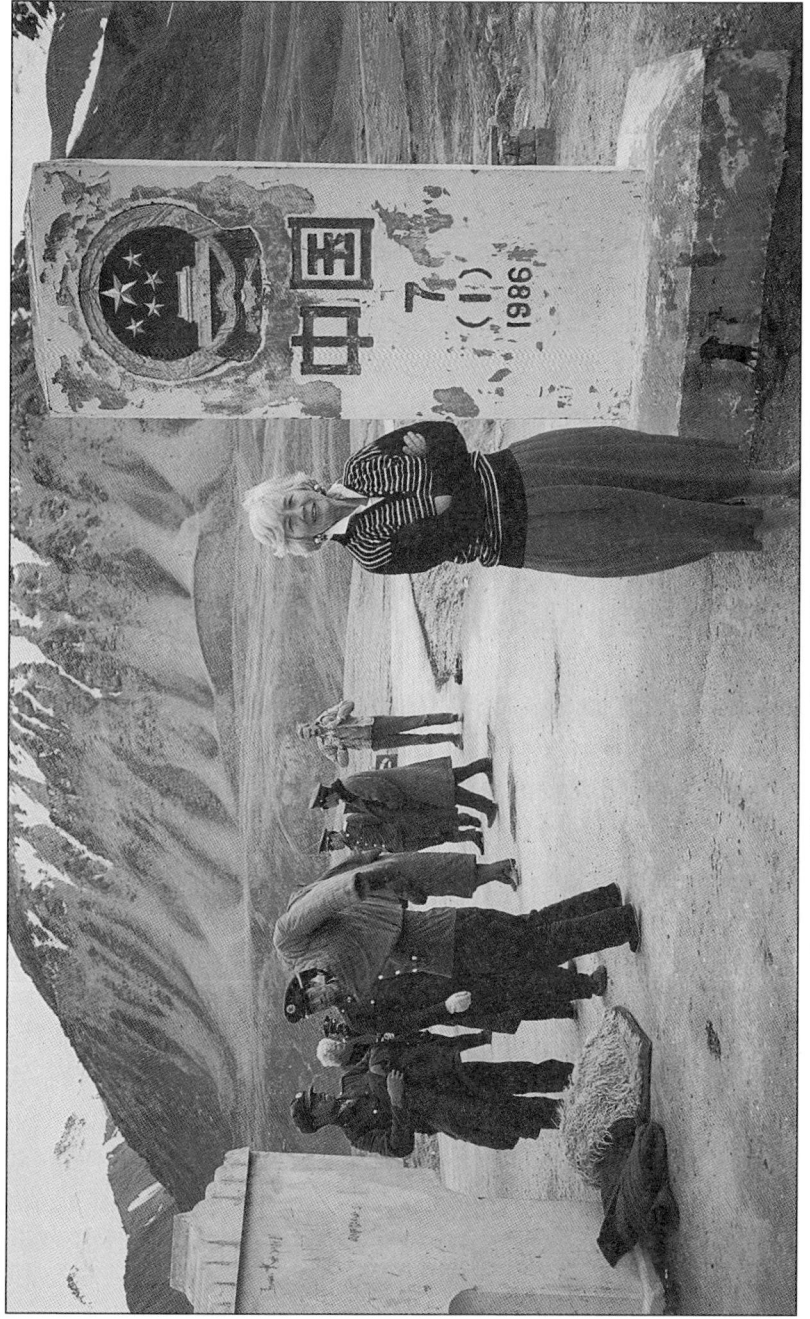

Jenny at Chinese border on Karakoram Highway

most warmly, and who had looked after them when taking postgraduate courses and examinations.

The formal visit was now over but five couples stayed on to make a private trip in a mini-bus up the Karakoram Highway, the old Chinese silk route, via Gilgit, Karimabad, Baltit and along the course of the River Indus and River Hunza to the Chinese border. In the Hunza Valley I could see the famous Hunza apricots drying on rooftops but as we went on we were overwhelmed with the sight of the mountainous Rakaposhi and Anna Purna peaks. At the Chinese border we had reached an altitude of 15,000 feet and sadly the five physicians had forgotten about acute mountain sickness! We had ascended the last 3 to 4,000 feet in our little bus very quickly. Fortunately morbidity was not too severe and we were able to return even more quickly. Those who had been disturbed by the altitude soon recovered and all was well.

This was our main College overseas expedition during my tcrm of office. However the President is normally invited to the English-speaking colleges all over the world and is usually honoured personally but this is, of course, an ex officio honour to the College. I had become a Fellow of the London College of Physicians the hard way. The Glasgow College and the Edinburgh College of Surgeons and the Dublin College kindly bestowed their Fellowships 'ad hominem'. However apart from Hon Fellowship of the College in Pakistan, Hon Fellowships were also granted by the American College at a meeting in San Francisco, the Australasian College in Sydney and the South African College at a meeting in Johannesburg. These and many other visits occasioned gatherings of Edinburgh Fellows, either indigenous citizens or migrants from the UK.

Air travel is often disturbed by the request over the loudspeaker, 'Is there a doctor on the plane?' Usually one is spared by some 'young blood' getting up to offer his services. I have, however, had a few personal experiences and there is always some concern lest it be something serious. The pilot may have to be asked to return to base or descend to an airport with access to a nearby hospital. I will recall only three episodes.

Once it was an elderly man lying flat out, semi-conscious and looking very pale and ill. His wife whispered in my ear, 'It's alright Doctor, he's had far too much to drink' – and she was right.

Another time we came down in Riyadh after I had been yet again to King Faisal University. It was late at night and shortly after taking off, dinner was served, and then the familiar request came over the air, 'Is there a doctor on the plane?' The concern was a young woman, a few rows behind me, who told me that she could not feel her arms or her legs and she felt very faint. I could see very little of her because she was dressed in traditional robes but she had a very distended leg almost certainly due to an old deep vein thrombosis and she was going to see a doctor in Harley Street. She said that she was sure her blood pressure had dropped and indeed I wondered if she might have had a pulmonary embolism. However, her pulse felt normal and her neck veins were not engorged. I said to the air hostess that if I could take the woman's blood pressure it might reassure my patient and certainly it would reassure me. This meant opening the medicine chest and after about fifteen minutes the hostess returned to say that the Captain wanted to be sure that I was a doctor. I told her to inform the Captain that if we did not get a move on my patient might slip away, and in my irritation I added that my dinner was getting cold! All was well, but the lady troubled me for reassurance all night. No doubt she was hysterical, and happily we arrived safely in London. I sometimes on reflection felt that I should have sent Saudi Airlines the fee that the Harley Street doctor would be charging!

A happier episode occurred on the long flight from Brisbane in Queensland home via Singapore. A few hours out of Brisbane, I was asked to see a little girl aged three who was crying with abdominal pain. I have no idea how the air hostess thought that I might be a doctor. I was able to make friends with the little girl and she let me examine her abdomen lying on pillows on the cabin floor. I felt reasonably sure that it was nothing serious like acute appendicitis, but I thought that she should be checked by the doctor in Singapore airport during our stopover there. She was given a half tablet of paracetamol and when I went back to see her, she was asleep in her mother's arms. The Chief Steward was anxious to give my wife some gifts by way of thanks and these were gratefully received. However, some time later I got a delightful letter of appreciation from Singapore Airlines to say that my little friend had arrived safely in Manchester and how grateful the airline and the family were to me. This had never happened to me before or since.

One other great privilege during the Presidency was invitations to many non-medical gatherings. These for me included such events as the annual dinners of the Writers to the Signet and the High Constables of Holyrood House. There was also a 175th anniversary celebration dinner for *The Scotsman* newspaper. This happened to be on Burns Night and the late John Smith proposed 'The Immortal

Memory' and Ian Lang, Secretary of State for Scotland proposed 'The Scotsman'. The famous fiddler Ally Bain was also there to give us some music. I remember his saying that he had been in Wick the previous evening and to his surprise, very few people in Wick seemed to have heard of *The Scotsman*, or of Ian Lang! Mr Lang took this in characteristically good part. Another annual event was to represent the College at the summer graduation at the Medical School. As we processed in and out behind the Principal, the College of Surgeons mace was twice as big as that leading the University Principal and ours was three times as big!

There were also many distinguished visitors to the College. Lord Mackay of Clashfern and HRH Princess Anne each received the Honorary Fellowship of our College, a very special distinction with only some twenty-five holders at any one time. Both spoke splendidly at the dinner gatherings celebrating their induction.

We also had a visit from Mrs Thatcher for a small non-medical dinner accompanied by Mr Lang, Mr Forsyth and Mr Rifkind. I was astonished to find that no Prime Minister in office had ever been in the College before – and she seemed to be most impressed with our history and our building. Mr Gladstone had had dinner in the Great Hall but that was when he was Chancellor of the Exchequer and had just been elected as Lord Rector in the University. Indeed we came across fascinating correspondence in the College archives from the Principal of the University asking courteously if the University might 'dine-in' Mr Gladstone in the Great Hall of the College. The President of the day had responded with a most 'shirty' letter to the effect that in these unusual circumstances the University could dine in

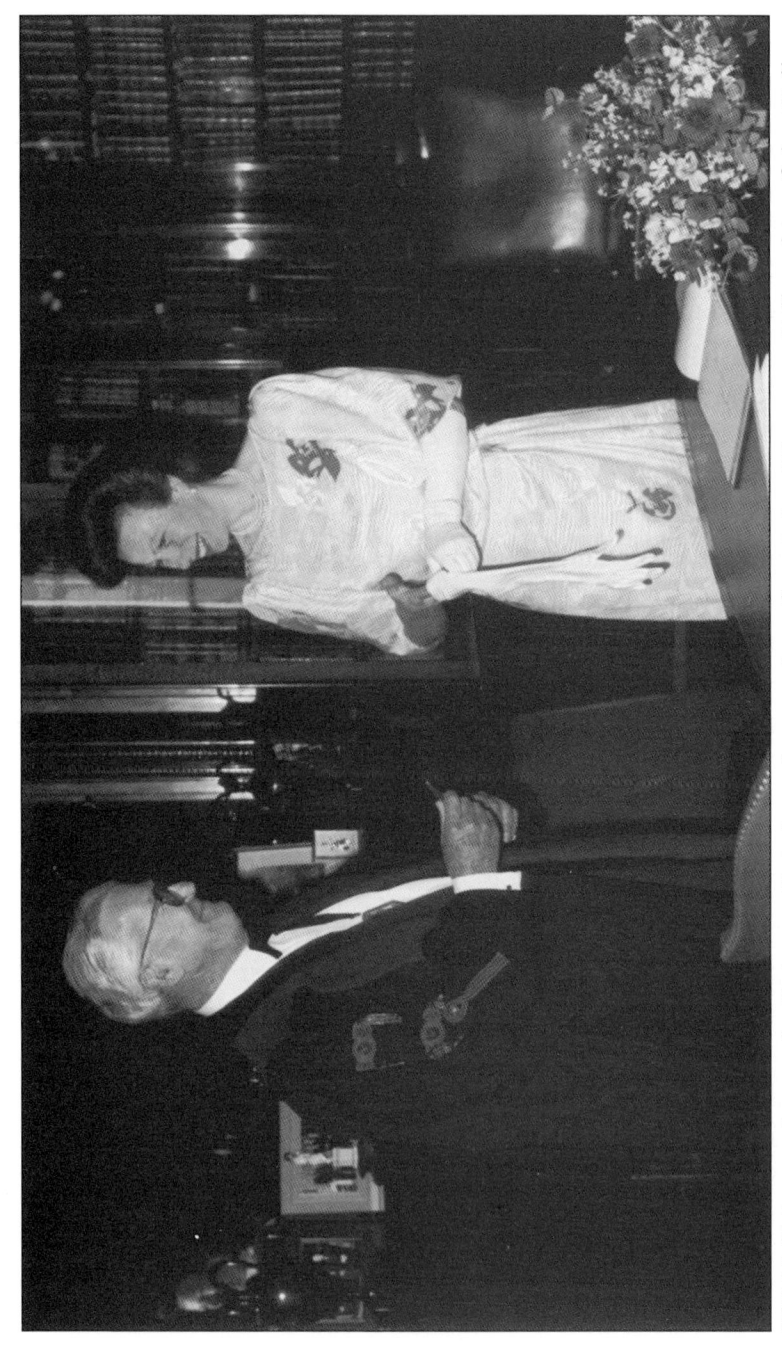

HRH Princess Anne, the Princess Royal on the evening of receiving Honorary Fellowship of the College. Signing the Visitor's Book in the President's Office.

the College but 'in no way was this to be construed as a precedent'! Mrs Thatcher enjoyed this also.

In 1990 the College held a symposium with an exhibition to commemorate the bicentenary of the death of past President William Cullen. In the University of Edinburgh he had been successively the Professor of Chemistry, of Physiology and then of Medicine. In the University Faculty he was the third Professor of Medicine after Rutherford and Gregory. In 1773-5 he was President of the College. He was a prominent figure among the personalities of the Scottish Enlightenment and Adam Smith and David Hume were his immediate friends. Boswell invited him to meet Dr Johnson at a small supper party on their brief visit to Edinburgh. Above all he was a great teacher and more than any other he was responsible for Edinburgh being the foremost medical school in the world of his day. Among his main contributions was to train a small group of pupils from the American colonies who were to found the first medical school in North America in Philadelphia (see Chapter 3). Among them was John Morgan who was to be the first Dean and Benjamin Rush a later signatory of the Declaration of Independence.

This influence of Cullen causes one to realise that Edinburgh's traditions were to originate in Padua and Leiden and apart from early contributions widely throughout the UK and in military medicine, a particular legacy seems to be that its emphasis on sound medical training and practice was to spread to America and then the Empire and Commonwealth. Interestingly, until recent years and the evolution of the European Community, our UK medical profession has had limited relationship with medicine in continental Europe.

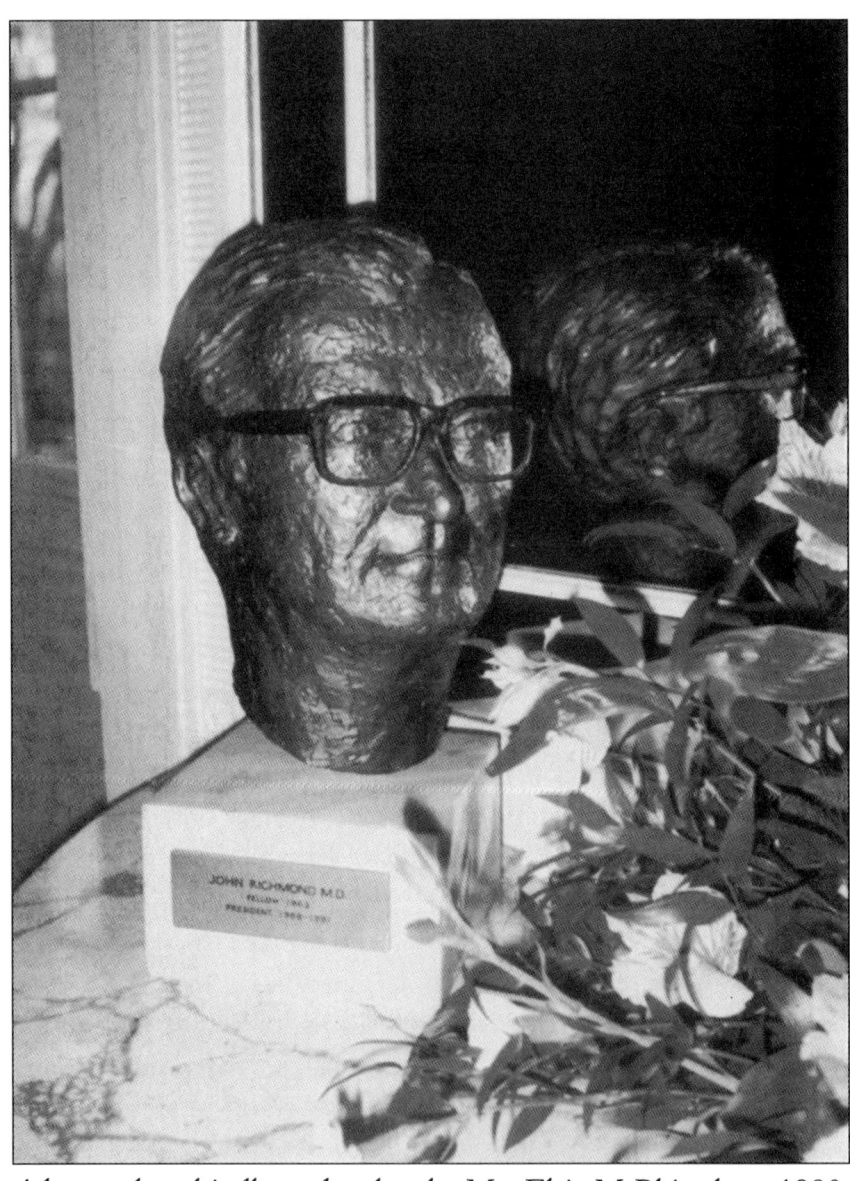

A bronze bust kindly undertaken by Mrs Elsie McPhie about 1980.
Mrs McPhie was the wife of our Church Elder in Sheffield. I was
much honoured to receive this and it now resides in the Davidson
Room (named after Sir Stanley Davidson) of the College.

Near the end of my time we learned that a painting in Spinks saleroom in St James in London by John Piper had been wrongly titled 'Old College University of Edinburgh' but was in fact the Royal College of Physicians of Edinburgh. Its origin is not accurately known but it was thought to have been bought by an American academic when in England and sold at auction in New York. We thought it essential that the painting should come to us and perhaps we could dedicate it to the memory of a past President, Dr Robertson, who had served the College faithfully over many years and who had recently died.

Happily we were able to purchase the picture and after a meeting in London I brought it to Edinburgh myself on a busy Friday evening starting off my journey standing all the way on the Underground with the picture between my legs from Piccadilly to Heathrow. I was greatly relieved to get home with no damage done.

Mr Piper was still alive and I took the liberty of writing to him to ask if he could remember any detail. Mrs Piper telephoned me on his behalf and although she could not recall this particular work she thought that it had probably been done when they had stayed with Professor Waddington in Edinburgh in 1951. I thought that I might learn a little more about Mr Piper in my Oxford Companion to Art. The tribute to him mentioned that in the late 1930s he had reverted to a 'romantic naturalism' and 'reverting to his early interest in architecture he painted topographical fantasies of great houses in decay'!

When I left Intake Junior Mixed School, even if I had been mature enough to contemplate the future, I could not have imagined in my wildest dreams that life's jigsaw would be made up of so many exciting pieces.

Just before demitting office as President I had one more rather moving duty and that was to represent the College at the St Andrew's Day service in the historic St Giles Cathedral and to read one of the lessons along with the Governor of Edinburgh Castle and GOC Scotland.

CHAPTER 10

Winding Down,
Retirement and Reflections

During a visit to Cape Town in November 2000, I began to think of a few possible topics for this final chapter. It was of course fifty years earlier that Jenny and I had met in Northern Rhodesia and I have already recounted how on my journey from Lusaka, then to Salisbury and finally to Cape Town our frequent correspondence had led to more than just friendship. When I boarded RMS *Stirling Castle* there was a cable awaiting Captain Richmond which I have to this day: 'Happy journey. Game definitely on. All love Jenny'.

The last ten years have of course been much different from the previous decades but nonetheless eventful. Compared with all the detail of professional life in earlier chapters what will follow is more concerned with random reflections, family, travelling and longstanding friendships.

The first thing that I realised was that it was important to 'get out of the hair' of my successor as President of the College. This was Dr Tony Toft who had been a very supportive Vice-President during my own term of office and he with his wife have been good friends. I have however kept an active interest in College affairs, particularly the frequent symposia, the Library and for the first six years I was one of the four trustees. Trusteeship is quite an important duty because the College with all its responsibilities for

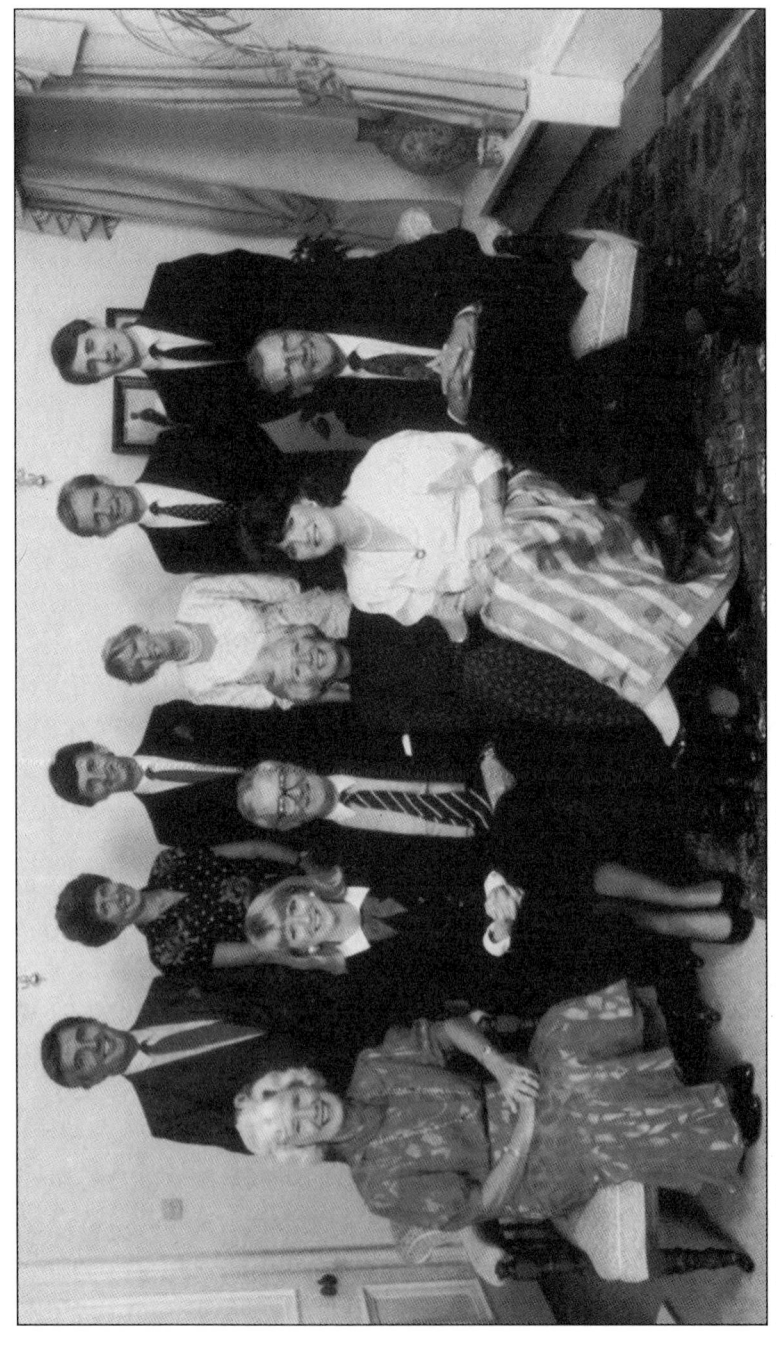

Ruby wedding celebration September 1991. Family gathering includes my brother and sister, our two sons and daughter and all the spouses. It was a lovely occasion.

examinations, continuing medical education (CME) and overseas links, is completely independent of government, its income arising mainly from Fellows' and Members' subscriptions and examination fees. Past presidents, of which there are now nine, meet for lunch usually three times per year.

From 1990-3, I served on the Department of Health Clinical Standards Advisory Group set up by Virginia Bottomley when she was Minister of Health. There were only eight of us in the group representing the main branches of Medicine; I was the physician and the one domiciled in Scotland. We had a non-medical chairman and lay secretary and our meetings were attended by the Chief Medical Officers of England, Scotland and Wales, the President of the General Medical Council and the President or Secretary of the Royal College of Nursing.

Our first survey was into 'Access to, and availability of, specialist services'. The sub-group with co-opted members for the survey looked at neonatal services, cystic fibrosis, childhood leukaemia and surgery for coronary artery disease, being a representative mixture of specialist subjects and I had the privilege of being the chairperson. We discovered a number of significant problems and geographical disparities and ended with strong recommendations.

Our report was presented independently and there was media interest. There followed a reasoned government reply. However I am not certain that things have changed very much since then. Indeed while I have been little involved over the years with this sort of central committee work, I did realise how time consuming and frustrating it could be. Since then I have come to fear that politics and the daily media attention could have an inhibiting effect on essential progress and definitive action.

Also in 1993 I was greatly honoured at New Year with notice of a CBE 'for services to academic medicine', which was awarded by HM The Queen at Holyrood Palace and then in summer 1994 with an Hon. MD in the University of Sheffield. Both led to happy family gatherings. I think that the first time I ever had cause to visit Holyrood Palace was to see our number one son receive the Duke of Edinburgh Gold Award from HRH Prince Philip himself. That would be in 1970.

Active interest in medical affairs never dies but 'hands on' clinical work becomes more and more unusual. Indeed the only duty which led to examination of patients (referred to as 'clients' or 'claimants') was participation in Medical Appeal Tribunals, which were served by a surgeon and physician and chaired by a lawyer. This went on until age seventy-two when one has to stand down.

However I have served for several years on the Scottish Committee of Marie Curie Cancer Care and also during a period as Chairman of the Professional Care Committee of the Marie Curie Centre in Edinburgh, the only other Marie Curie Hospice in Scotland being in Glasgow. In addition there are several hundred Marie Curie nurses scattered throughout Scotland giving 'hands on' care. It has been splendid to see the great and long overdue evolution of palliative medicine and the marvellous teamwork of doctors, nurses, physiotherapists, occupational therapists, social workers, homecare sisters and religious advisors as well as the great support given selflessly by lay volunteers.

Evolution in the community is also taking place and so is undergraduate medical student training. Apart from the Marie Curie hospices there are seven others in Scotland, including a Children's hospice, all largely dependent on

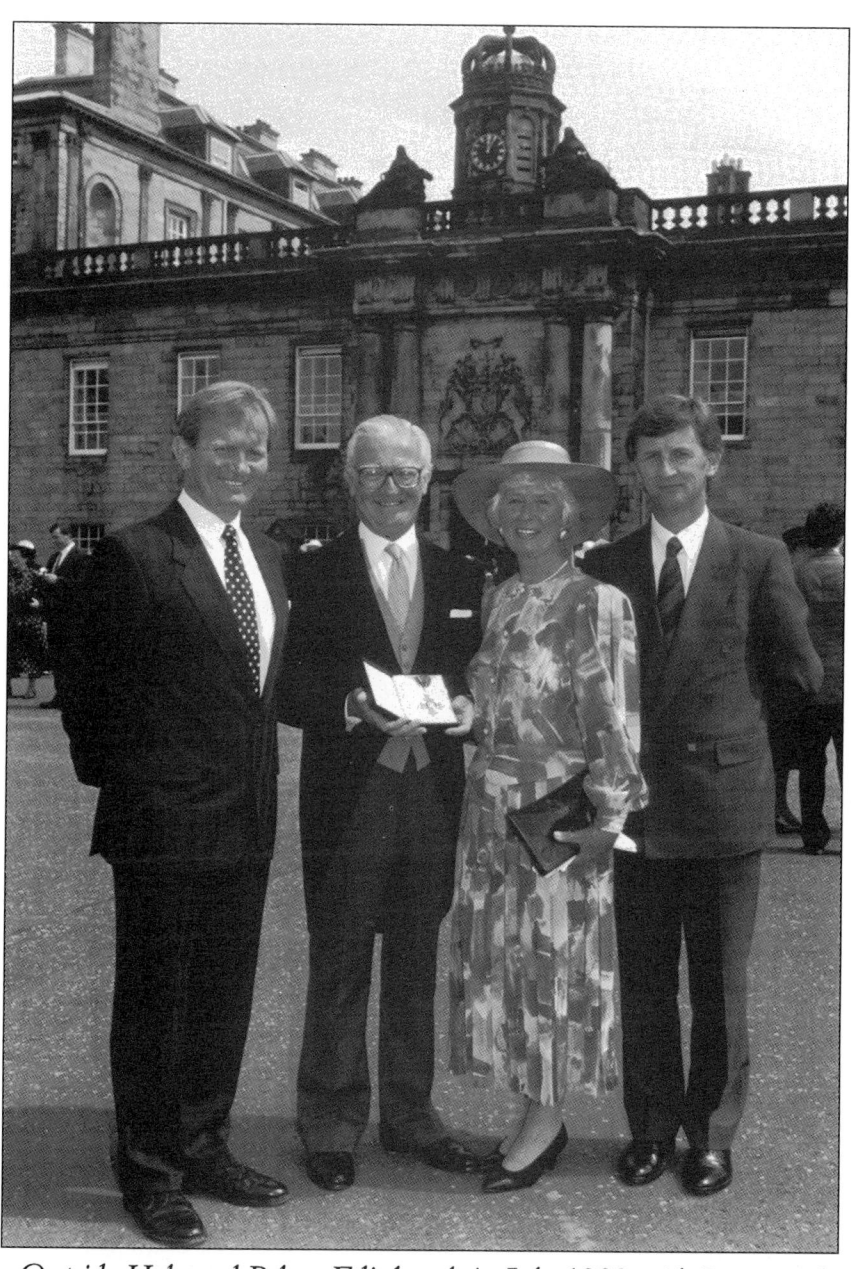

*Outside Holyrood Palace Edinburgh in July 1993 with Jenny and
two sons after being awarded the CBE.*

charity. Before leaving the subject of palliative medicine, I have to emphasise the enormous importance of the nursing profession's role and contribution.

I served for some six years on the Scottish Advisory Committee of the British Council as the only medical person. The British Council is of course one of our major national institutions providing support all over the world and attracting many foreign students here. I look back with some amusement at my first encounter in 1949 during my period of National Service in Addis Ababa. I was invited one evening to attend a British Council occasion and the main event was to watch the teaching of the local Amharas how to do Morris Dancing!

From 1994-6 I served part-time as Vice Dean in the Edinburgh University Faculty of Medicine. This was another period of meeting old friends and treading over old ground and bringing back happy memories. One thing that did strike me during this spell in the Medical School, and of course not for the first time, was the emphasis on the very high academic qualifications required of student applicants to Medical Schools nowadays before they can even be considered for a place.

As is widely known throughout the country, selection for a Medical School requires A grades in 'A' levels and in Scottish Highers, the more the better. We do of course need high fliers in Medicine but not everyone should need to have multiple A grades. I may be in danger of causing offence but it is so important to remember that most branches of Medicine need compassion, ability to listen, communication skills and patience. I feel strongly that all potential candidates, and that may mean 500-600 in most medical schools, should be interviewed; this we used to do in Edinburgh in years gone by and also in Sheffield. Usually the interviewers were in pairs and it takes a little practice to put a naturally apprehensive candidate at his or her ease. One also has to make personal adjustment if interviewing an assured public school student followed by a crofter's son or daughter from the Outer Isles. However, even in relatively short interviews I have the strong feeling that one can get an impression of the applicants who might make good doctors. Perhaps we should look at interviewing again although it is yet another time-consuming exercise.

Another thought about University medicine which goes back to my Sheffield days is the increasing burden of administration and fiscal control. Indeed in order for medical schools to survive and prosper these days, it is becoming more important to attract staff with research expertise who will bring in research funding, perhaps at the expense of bringing in staff whose main contribution would be in teaching.

In retirement and semi-retirement one has to keep out of one's wife's way, except to give more domestic support than previously. But also our social life assumes increasing importance. Returning to old friendships in Edinburgh has been delightful; also we have been blessed with nice neighbours. The present house is in the same general area as earlier ones and near good shops and buses into town. We are even within bath chair distance of the nearby super-market.

I, and sometimes Jenny is able to accompany me, get happy outings to the Senior Fellows Clubs in the Colleges of Physicians and of Surgeons. Both have monthly lunch-time gatherings over the winter period, with most interesting and varied lectures.

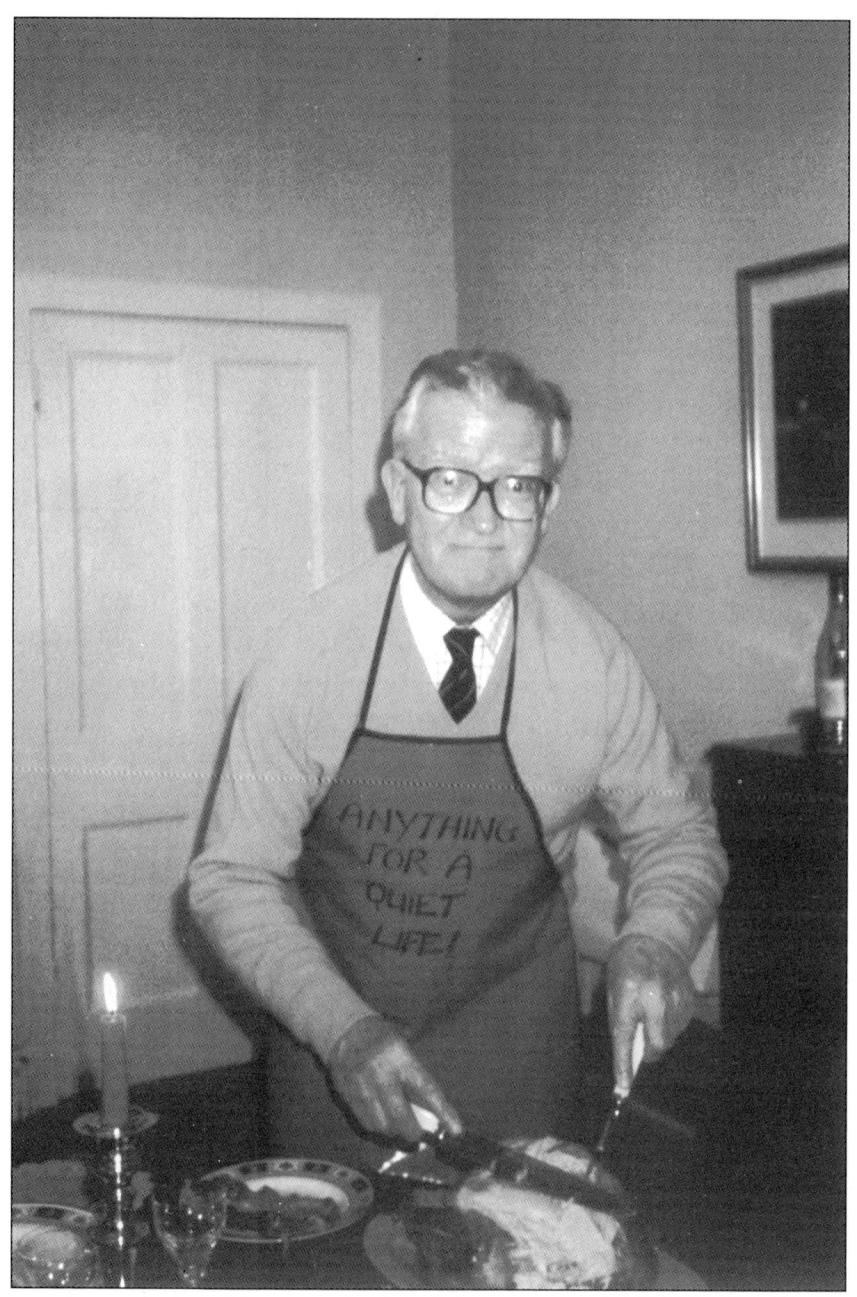

Trying to be helpful in retirement.

I belong to a group of Medical Pilgrims which was founded in 1927. A few physicians from the main medical centres meet annually at different University sites and sometimes overseas, usually in May. The gatherings last for two or three days and combine a scientific meeting, a visit to some local place of historic interest and a couple of dinners. Being 'pilgrims' we are supposed to dress sparingly and eat frugally but nothing could be further from the truth. In a recent history of the Medical Pilgrims which puts together all the Scribes' Minutes, I note that in 1954 in Edinburgh:

> At morning coffee the news came that Stanley Davidson who had appeared fit at dinner the previous evening was unable to give his analysis of an impressive series of patients with macrocytic anaemia, but Dr John Richmond stepped into the breach at short notice with much ability!

I had the great honour of being leader in Cambridge in 1992. Our main dinner was in Christ's College and we had many distinguished guests. I was seated between our host, the Master, Sir Hans Kornberg, who began his career as a laboratory technician with the great Hans Krebs in Sheffield in the early 1930s, and Lord Todd of Trumpington who chaired the Royal Commission on Medical Education (the Todd Report), of 1968, to which I referred in Chapter 7. This was to have enormous importance and influence in the 1970s and subsequently.

I also greatly enjoy membership of the Aesculapian Club, which goes back to the eighteenth century and is believed to be the longest continually functioning dining club in the world. There are eleven physicians and eleven surgeons and we meet twice yearly in the Royal College of Physicians along with our guests. We also have a distinguished principal guest and when it was my turn to be in the Chair we had Lord Wilson of Tillyorn, the penultimate Governor of Hong Kong.

I must not omit mentioning membership of the Edinburgh Corner Club. This is a very mixed social group mostly of retirees chaired by a one-time paper maker and including a banker, mathematician, electroplater, pharmacologist, architect, advertiser and two other doctors. We meet in a local hostelry and share reminiscences and much good humour.

In 1998 we had a 50th reunion of the Edinburgh 1948 medical graduates (my class), and it was another memorable occasion. Some seventy of the class were able to attend along with sixty spouses and they came from as far away as Vancouver and Tasmania, as well as Cape Town, other parts of North America and the Antipodes. We started with a relaxed buffet gathering in the New Club on Princes Street with its unique panoramic outlook towards the Castle. Next morning we had a few light-hearted papers in the Old College of the University (where we had taken most of our examinations). Then lunch with the Dean in the Playfair Library. The evening dinner which rounded off the gathering was in the Great Hall of the College of Physicians. As I have felt at previous reunions, most of the men were looking a little older but the women all looked more alluring than I remembered them from student days!

Perhaps the greatest enjoyment in retirement and when winding down is good holidays, often with friends. I have already had cause to mention travelling widely during University and Colleges of Physicians' appointments. Although these trips were excellent there would always be some important duties as part of them. Now it is all about relaxing, seeing places of interest not so far visited, although we go back frequently to some venues, and hoping to find good weather.

We went many times in years gone by, but not lately, to Gozo by Malta and the Algarve. I think that our main trips in recent years have been to southern Africa, to Australia and to France.

The visits to southern Africa have been largely for family reasons, but it is also a lovely country and such a tragedy that there is so much uncertainty about the future. In the middle of the 1990s Jenny and I made one trip to central Africa, where our happy life together had started. We went first to Harare in Zimbabwe where one gained the impression then of peace and prosperity. Then back to Lusaka where we stayed with old and dear farming friends. Zambia seemed desperate. I have already mentioned how in 1950 there were very few doctors there but now there is a 1,500-bed teaching hospital in which on my visit I was distressed to find that so many of the patients had Aids. Our next stop was the Victoria Falls Hotel, the original one. The Falls was my last stop on the recruiting trip recounted in Chapter 4, when I could not return to Lusaka quickly enough to meet up with my new lady.

France is an almost annual holiday and in recent years we have gone mostly to Grimaud in Provence, the old village just inland from St Tropez, where we rent a delightful cottage from friends. Usually we drive all the way, perhaps going south through the Loire Valley and back through places like Chablis and Epernay.

Earlier in my story I have spoken of research in haematology and the spleen. On leaving Sheffield it was customary for the 'has beens' to give a lecture on something which colleagues might not know had given much interest in the past. 'Secrets of the spleen' was perfect.

Nearer the time of the lecture I discovered a claret which seemed to be well regarded, known as 'Chateau Chasse-Spleen' and I thought that a picture of a bottle would make a good last lantern slide. Then I thought that it would be a good idea to know what 'Chasse-Spleen' meant. The Professor of French was not much help because 'chasse' means 'the chase' or 'the hunt'. Then more or less fortuitously I discovered that the owner of the vineyard in Moulis-en-Medoc was a young widow and I wrote to her with my problem. She responded with a very nice letter including a picture of herself in front of the Chateau and permission to use this as my very last slide. The letter went on to say that I was not anywhere near the answer. Charles Baudelaire had enjoyed the claret on one particularly sad day and suggested the name 'Chasse-Spleen'. 'Chasse' comes from the verb 'chasser', 'to chase' or 'to send away', and in French, spleen is the word for melancholy. 'Chasse-Spleen' is therefore to send away the melancholy, and so it does! I have since had a most enjoyable visit to the chateau and to meet the helpful lady.

Not surprisingly we have much enjoyed Australia. There were two official visits in the Edinburgh College days but several subsequent visits have been for good holidays. One in the early 1990s had an unusual background. Jenny and I had been considering a trip to Johannesburg to see her older sister and husband around Christmas time. An Edinburgh friend (and old classmate) Douglas Bell, President of the University Union in 1947-8, hearing of this, asked if there was any chance of our going to Sydney for one of his daughter's weddings which had been arranged on a date

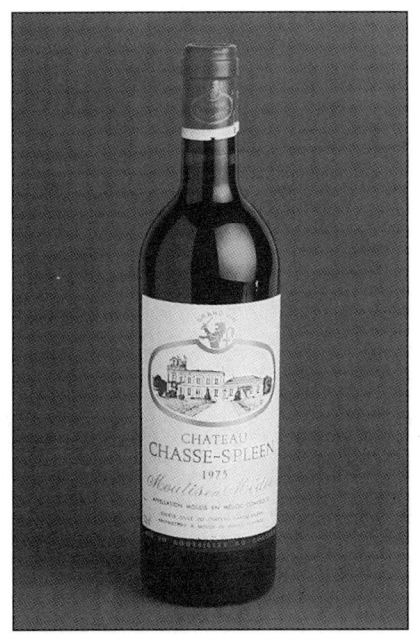

A bottle of Chateau Chasse-Spleen.

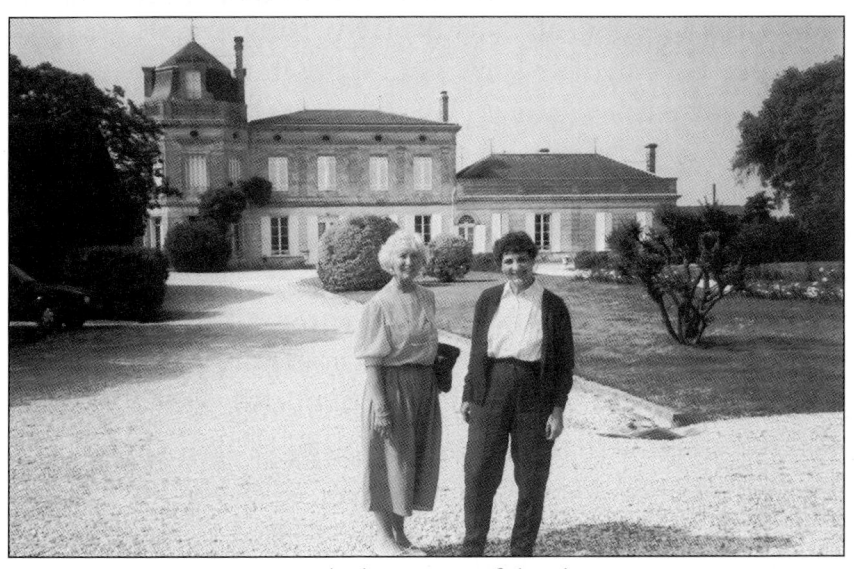

Jenny with the owner of the chateau.

between Christmas and New Year. Well Sydney and Johannesburg are not exactly close to each other geographically but of course we said 'Yes'. The daughter had actually been best maid at our own daughter's wedding.

We ended up spending Christmas in Fiji after a long journey via Los Angeles and Honolulu. Crossing the date line on Jenny's birthday meant that it lasted for only six hours! We had a delightful Christmas celebration in Fiji with local children singing carols in candlelight before going on to Sydney for the wedding. Then we joined another old classmate and his wife for a memorable New Year's Eve gathering. The midnight fireworks were of course spectacular which causes me to mention the unique and outstanding displays of the Olympics 2000.

Next day we had a marvellous outing sailing round Sydney Harbour and meeting up with another old classmate, after which we travelled on to South Africa before returning home to the cold of Edinburgh.

The last time in Australia before writing this also had its memorable events. We stayed primarily in the Brisbane area where Jenny has relatives. We drove down to Sydney and had a few days in a nice hotel overlooking Circular Quay and one morning looking out of our window had the glorious spectacle of the QE2 coming in between the Opera House and the Harbour Bridge.

After returning to Brisbane we went on to a holiday place known as Noosa Heads, about two hours drive northwards. This time we did not do the Barrier Reef which we had enjoyed on an earlier trip, but stayed in recommended and so-called 'luxury apartments' known as 'On The Beach', and they were. The apartments were serviced by contract cleaners and on our penultimate day the cleaning lady in conversation mentioned that she was having trouble with her eyes and was going to receive laser treatment; however her doctor was being very cautious. I said that he must be Scottish, but she said that he was not Scottish, and she thought he had trained in some medical school in the middle of England. After some hesitation and thought she said, 'I am sure that it was a place called Sheffield'!

A little later the same doctor phoned because he was a graduate from around the middle of my time there and invited us round in the evening for drinks. Shortly after the phone went again and it was his wife inviting us round for dinner. She had been a young ward sister in the Royal Hallamshire Hospital. We did of course have a delightful evening with them.

Before leaving, the doctor said that he would like to show me his room in their lovely new house near Noosa Heads. It was a billiard room, full of books, but perhaps the most intriguing thing for me was his very large collection of old cameras. I went on to tell him that I had a few cameras and mostly used the inexpensive recent automatic ones. However at one time my great joy had been a Kodak Retina three 'c' which I had bought in New York in the late 1950s, and which had been stolen in a burglary. I was never able to replace it because it seemed to be little available in Britain. He asked was it a big 'C' or a little 'c'. I had to say that I could not remember. Then he produced a Retinette, a Retina I, a Retina II, a Retina III C and IIIc. I said that I was sure that it had been a big C. As we were leaving he said that he had actually got two big Cs and he gave me one. I felt very embarrassed but of course delighted; he added that he and his wife felt so grateful to Sheffield.

There is a danger of rambling on about these happy

memories. Like other contemporaries many of us have been greatly privileged. I often say that the furthest place my father had been able to travel to was the Isle of Man but that was how it was and as I have mentioned earlier, sadly he died rather early.

So much has happened in the last fifty years and the growth of knowledge and technology has been exponential. The growth has been remarkable in all things relating to medicine, and I realise how quickly I am getting out of touch in the short time that I have been retired. One has to wonder what will happen in the next fifty years. When in a long queue recently waiting for the computer to stop misbehaving my neighbour commented that things were much better in the 'carrier pigeon' era!

At the risk of indulging in too much nostalgia, I have to repeat my great indebtedness over the years to my school teachers and to the many who guided and influenced me so significantly in my medical education and subsequent development. I do not want to pick out individuals because I was in the care of many remarkable people. I also have to pay tribute to special and long-lasting friendships. Many were contemporaries in my medical school days and who themselves have made major contributions to all branches of medicine. Not only have they been very supportive of me but the happiest part of these friendships is that our wives all get on well together.

Our two sons and our daughter are all doctors and in active practice. As in many other families we have had some problems that we wish had not occurred. The lovely ten grandchildren are all doing well. The sequence is one girl, eight boys and one girl. I took the youngest three (two boys and a girl) to the Cinderella pantomime in Edinburgh at

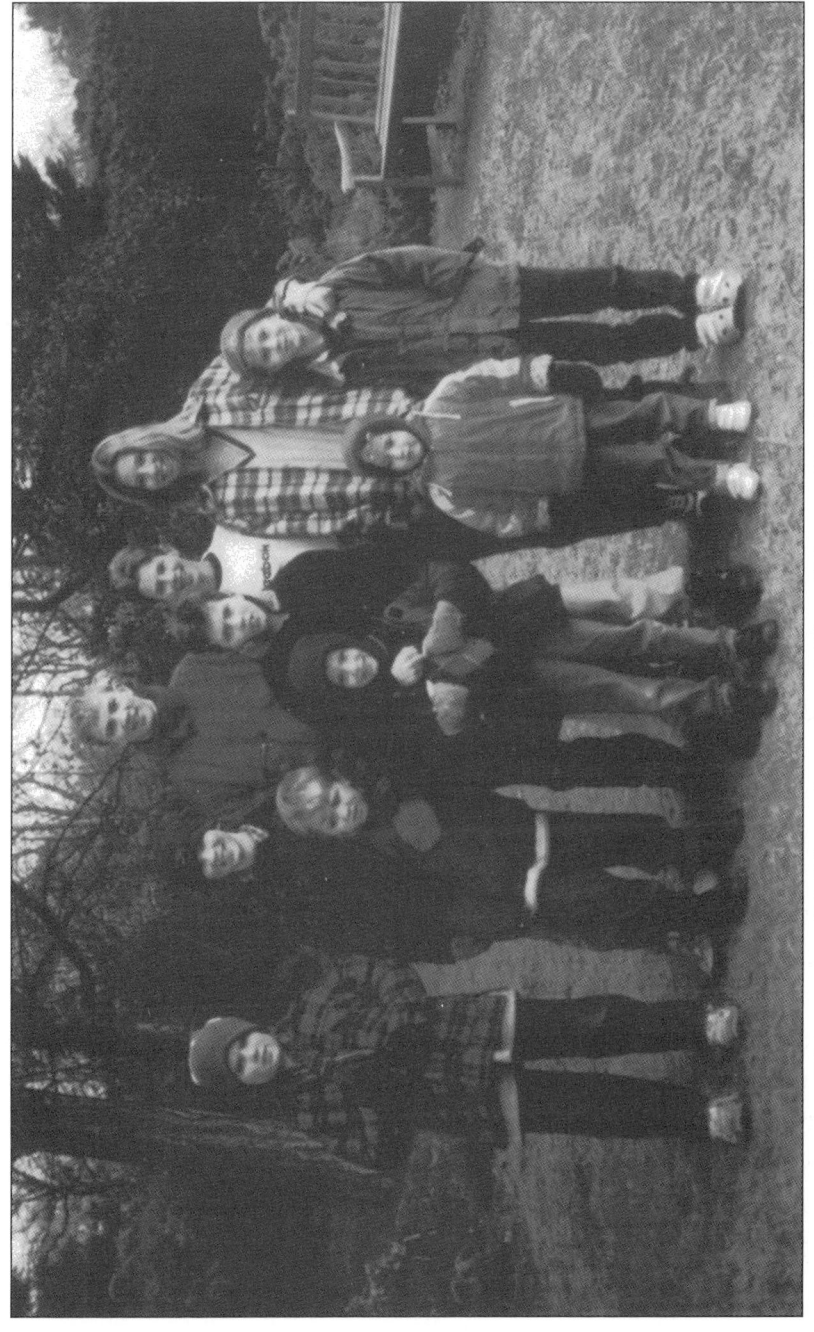

The ten grandchildren about to go hill walking on Boxing Day 1998.

159

New Year 2000. At the end of the show the granddaughter, then aged seven, was on the stage and seemed to outdo Buttons with her confident exchanges. When Buttons offered to be her boyfriend Daisy replied 'No way' and Buttons had to say that that was twice he had been turned down that evening. Also during this visit the children had Jenny and me playing games. One involved writing down a well-known name on a piece of paper. None of us could guess the name that Daisy had chosen. Although the spelling was not perfect, it was Slobodan Milosevic!

The older granddaughter has been on Operation Raleigh to Brunei and then followed with a teaching visit to Vietnam. She has a place at Cambridge to read Medicine, a change of heart she reached personally while in Brunei. Number two, the first grandson, also managed to get into Operation Raleigh and went to Chile at the same time as Prince William. The second part of his gap year was to assist with the teaching of sport and physical education in a school in North Queensland, Australia. His university place is at Manchester to read French and European Studies.

And so as I look back on my life I realise that it all just happened. I reflect particularly on how I came to meet Jenny and also on my first few years as a doctor. As I have already recounted, two of us were looking after a small but busy acute hospital, then I travelled through Africa, often in remote places alone as a doctor, before being thrust into a single-handed general practice miles from anywhere. Very fortunately no disasters occurred but in youthful confidence and ignorance one does not expect any. However, no young graduate nowadays would feel comfortable coping with that sort of responsibility. The undergraduate medical curriculum has been so much revamped over the years that there is now much fragmentation of what used to be the core subjects and there is early emphasis on specialism. We are needing to graduate 'basic doctors' as was the case in years gone by, more than ever. Specialism can follow later.

The acute hospitals are becoming increasingly broken up into specialties and hospital bed numbers nationwide are seriously crumbling. Care for the convalescent and long-term sick is increasingly difficult and the role of the 'family doctor', the personal one-to-one doctor has had to change also. We face much difficulty, but like others, I feel in my bones that a good, caring, generous Health Service is the core of a happy and successful society.

I conclude by saying that I have much enjoyed tracing the many pieces of life's jigsaw. But life is a jigsaw without a frame and it seems to extend in all directions.